the Grim Reaper's road map

An atlas of mortality in Britain

Mary Shaw, Bethan Thomas,

George Davey Smith and Daniel Dorling

First published in Great Britain in 2008 by

The Policy Press
University of Bristol
Fourth Floor, Beacon House
Queen's Road
Bristol BS8 1QU
UK

Tel +44 (0)117 331 4054
Fax +44 (0)117 331 4093
e-mail tpp-info@bristol.ac.uk
www.policypress.org.uk

© The Policy Press 2008

British Library Cataloguing in Publication Data
A catalogue record for this book is available from the British Library

Library of Congress Cataloging-in-Publication Data
A catalog record for this book has been requested

ISBN 978 1 86134 824 1 paperback
ISBN 978 1 86134 823 4 hardcover

Mary Shaw is an Honorary Research Fellow in the Department of Social Medicine, University of Bristol. **Bethan Thomas** and **Daniel Dorling** work in the Social and Spatial Inequalities Research Group in the Department of Geography at the University of Sheffield. **George Davey Smith** works in the Department of Social Medicine at the University of Bristol.

Cover design by The Policy Press, Bristol.
Front cover: image kindly supplied by www.alamy.com
Printed and bound in Great Britain by Latimer Trend, Plymouth.

For Mary, Tom and Lily Wells, and new beginnings

Contents

ACKNOWLEDGEMENTS

David Dorling, for his careful reading and insightful comments on an earlier draft. Paul Norman at the School of Geography, the University of Leeds, for the revised 'Estimating with Confidence' 1991 population figures. Ben Wheeler for acting as photographer's assistant at Arnos Vale Cemetery, Bristol. All the team at The Policy Press for their unstinting patience and support.

Mortality data for England and Wales were supplied by the Office for National Statistics, and for Scotland by the General Register Office for Scotland.

Digital boundaries are Crown Copyright and reproduced with the permission of the Controller of HMSO and the Queen's Printer for Scotland. Digital boundaries were obtained from then Census Geography Data Unit (UKBORDERS), EDINA (University of Edinburgh).

Plates on pages 2, 4, 18, 26, 152 and 190 are from *Human Physiology* by William Furneaux, revised by William A.M. Smart (Longmans, Green and Co, 1931). Plates on pages 20, 30, 94, 96, 122, 130, 132, 138, 158, 160, 166, 170, and 194 are from *Human Physiology* by John Thornton, revised by William A.M. Smart (Longmans, Green and Co, 1932). Plates on pages 40, 82 and 168 are from *Home Cyclopaedia of Popular Medical, Social & Sexual Science* by E.B. Foote (Murray Hill Pub Co, c1901). Plates on pages 44, 92 and 134 are from *Harmsworth's Home Doctor & Encyclopaedia of Good Health*, Volume 2 (Harmsworth's Encyclopaedias, c1925). Plate on page 188 is from http:// en.wikipedia.org/wiki/Image:EMpylori.jpg. In all cases permission to use the plates has been sought.

The maps on the inside covers show the location of some cities and towns on both the cartogram and a conventional map as an aid to navigation.

Introduction

1 What this book is about

This is an atlas of death. On these pages we show how death came to people on one small island over the course of some 24 years. Death comes to us all, but at different times and in different forms. When records of all deaths are brought together, patterns can be seen across the land. Each of our individual deaths cannot be predicted with great accuracy. However, collectively, mortality rates and variation by cause are known to be strongly patterned, according to our age, sex, when and where we were born, where we have moved to, the jobs we have done or not done, rewards we did or did not receive, and all the myriad environmental, social and economic 'insults' and benefits that our minds and bodies have suffered or rejoiced in. The understanding and depiction of the Grim Reaper's travels here uses ideas and methods drawn from medical sociology, computer cartography, clinical epidemiology and health geography. Understanding a little about these perspectives will enhance your understanding of what this atlas shows, and that is what the introduction to this book is about.

The book does not show simple or conventional maps. On a simple map of mortality most people will have died in those towns and cities where most people live, particularly in the places where there are more elderly people. This, however, is not an atlas for undertakers who need to know where the greatest numbers of people die. It *is* an atlas for those interested in the health of us all, including those who have died in the recent past and those who have many years left to go. Because we are interested in all people of all ages living in Britain, the maps used here are all population cartograms, where the projection used scales area so that each town and city in Britain is drawn roughly in proportion to its resident population while remaining located in roughly the right place on the map in relation to other places in Britain. We say 'roughly' twice here because we have also ensured that the maps show simple geometric shapes to aid legibility and to make the maps comparable to other atlases we have drawn.

Just as we have standardised geographical space in this atlas so that an even distribution of the population is produced, so too we have standardised by age and sex when calculating the mortality ratios used to colour these maps. What every map in this atlas shows is a person's chances of dying from a particular cause in a particular place compared with the national average chance for that cause of death, having standardised for the varying distributions of the population by age and sex in each area. Women constitute a higher proportion of the population in some parts of Britain than other parts and so you might expect people in those parts to live a little longer; women tend to live about 6 years longer than men. These factors are even more important when considering the differing risks and causes of death associated with particular ages. We give details of how the mortality ratios shown here were standardised in the Technical Appendix.

Because we map the standardised mortality ratio (SMR) for each neighbourhood, the maps do not show, for example, where more elderly people live or equally where fewer elderly people live. Also, death rates from one cause in one place will not appear low due to many people there dying from other causes. It would be theoretically possible for a dreadful place – the Grim Reaper's favourite visiting spot – to have high standardised mortality ratios for every condition mapped here. Such a place would have a much lower than average life expectancy. There are places in Britain where rates of dying from nearly all of the most significant causes of death are indeed elevated; where these places are becomes apparent as you look at the maps. Similarly there are places where death comes far later in most people's lives. To reiterate: places highlighted on these maps are thus not highlighted due to the age and sex profile of the population in each neighbourhood, but from death rates being higher or lower than expected for its population.

What causes death rates to vary from place to place? When asked this question people often suggest genetic factors. When genetic factors affect a condition, often a large number of different genes are involved, and within Britain relatively few genetic variants show consistent geographical gradients. It is likely that very few of our maps reflect different genetic distributions in different parts of the UK. The population of the UK is a vast genetic mix. People have moved over time between the cells drawn on these maps. What causes most of the variation shown on these maps are not factors inherent in the population living in each area, but external, environmental factors. There are many different types of environmental factor. Some are called lifestyle factors, a term which suggests some personal choices which are alterable by education. Our behaviour to a large degree is determined by our environments, such as whether those we live and work with smoke, drink and exercise. Some environmental factors affect all or most people in the locality, some just those in particular occupations or who engage in particular activities. Environmental factors not only affect the likelihood of a condition, but also the outcome. If treatment is sufficiently better in one place than another, you may be likely to live a year or two longer: that is unlikely to show up on the map. But if variations in treatment make you more likely to live than to die, that will affect these statistics.

Which environmental factors matter most has varied over the course of our recent history in Britain. In the distant past, living in areas more visited by plague, or where harvests were more variable, was most detrimental. When large numbers of people first began to mix in cities, rates of death from infectious disease rose sharply, killing huge numbers of babies in infancy. Under half a century ago, maps of mortality reflected mainly the risks of working in particularly regionally concentrated industries, absolute poverty and hunger, while the diseases of the affluent were caused, among other things, by their greater propensity at that time to smoke and eat rich diets. The most important underlying environmental factor today is *relative* poverty. It affects so many different and important causes that it alone is the most significant cause of the appearance of the map of 'All deaths' (see Map 1). Where more people are poor, they may no longer be hungry or thin, but many more die young than where the population is better off. Death rates are higher in general where people are poorer, especially where severe poverty is more common. A final factor has played a significant role in sharpening up these geographical differences in recent decades: migration.

At the start of the period for which deaths are being mapped here, the country suffered its greatest economic recession since that of the 1930s. Mass unemployment came to Britain in the early 1980s but affected some places far more than others. A government minister at the time suggested that if people wanted work they could 'get on their bikes' to find it, just as millions did in the '30s. Many did move around the country with their families looking for jobs. However, their chances of gaining those jobs were not all equal. Those with a little more going for

them did, on average, better in the labour market, got on the housing ladder and moved out of poorer areas. Those whose lives were a little harder to start with found themselves more often left in places that the more fortunate had left. The country became dramatically polarised between rich and poor, north and south, inner city and affluent suburb, idyllic rural village and concrete ghost town. Between 1950 and 1980 the geographical and social divides had narrowed, but over the period drawn here they widened sharply.

One result of social geographical polarisation was that different parts of Britain became increasingly areas more for the poor or areas more for the rich. When this happens it becomes more important where you live if you want access to a peaceful environment, 'good' schools, an efficient health service, well-rewarded work, good quality housing and so on. More and more often, people who could do so moved out of areas that were falling down the relative social scales. More and more often, people living in affluent areas who lost their jobs, or whose relationships failed, found that they had to move to less desirable locations to find cheaper housing. In the recent past there had been some cheaper housing in most places. During the 1980s and 1990s it became concentrated mainly in the poorest parts of towns and cities and in poorer rural areas.

Social inequalities resulting in geographical polarisation occur throughout the life course. The sons and daughters of the rich might spend part of their lives living in student ghettos. The right-to-buy of council housing has resulted in almost no state housing in many rural and affluent enclaves. Developers have built differently sized and priced homes for sale in different places according to exact measures of what it is thought the market will bear for each location. Where there was no space for building, but incomes were high, older homes were renovated and made more expensive mainly by cosmetic changes and through fashion. And just as we store up environmental 'insults' and benefits to our health over time, so we store up financial debt or wealth and geographically live in very different places in old age according to our economic fortunes. As a result, we die at different rates and of differing causes in different places.

All human life comes to an end and all that affects human life affects that end. Here we have concentrated on providing a description of how the country looks when deaths from a period of 24 years are used to colour its surface. We provide a little detail on all deaths and major groups of causes of death first. Next we show which causes of death are most common in which places at what ages. Then, in the bulk of the book each of the causes we identify is described and mapped, and some brief suggestions are offered as to why each map looks like it does. There are two maps if we find the maps for males and females differ sufficiently for separate maps to be shown.

After mapping all deaths, we map nine groups of causes of deaths: all cardiovascular causes, all cancers, all transport-related deaths, and so on. *We have ordered the maps by the order of average age at death for each group.* There then follow 99 categories of death which encompass all possible causes of death. *Again, the order is that of the average age at death for each category.* Some of these categories are single causes, such as prostate cancer, while others are combinations of related causes of death, such as endocrine disorders (excluding diabetes). As the bulk of death registrations for the time period covered in this atlas used the ninth revision of the International Classification of Diseases (ICD), this was the version we used in designing our categories. There are, of course, many possible combinations that we could have chosen. Some of the categories are in themselves simple and obvious: the various types of cancer, for instance. The various methods of suicides and undetermined causes – where open verdicts have been returned by the coroner (or in Scotland, the procurator fiscal) – have been put into single categories. Heart attacks and chronic heart disease were put into one category: this will cover numerous possible entries on the death certificate.

The 99 categories of cause of death which we map are ordered by average age at death, starting at the lowest age. We present for each cause: the total number of cases over the time period (1981 to 2004); the percentage of all deaths that this cause accounts for; the average age of death; and the male to female ratio of the number of deaths. At the end of this introduction we list how many millions of years of life have been lost by people dying from each cause from not living to the age of 75.

The maps in this atlas have not been seen before. They show patterns that are in many cases quite different to maps drawn by previous generations of cartographers of causes of death. Some may inspire researchers to search for new ideas about why the patterns are as they are. Others may inspire readers to think of how these patterns might look in the future across this island when their own death records, those of whom they love, and of all their near and more distant neighbours are each making a slight contribution to the particular colouring of just one particular pixel on one place on just one map – yet to be drawn. We hope that many of the maps will encourage you to reflect on how unfair life often is, even in a prosperous country.

2 Location maps

We have used population cartograms to map the causes of death in this atlas. Population cartograms map each area according to the size of its population. The centres of cities, which are almost indistinguishable on a conventional map, become visible on the cartogram, while the rural parts of Britain, which cover a large area on the ground but are sparsely populated, are reduced in size on the cartogram. Each parliamentary constituency is represented as a hexagon on the maps that follow. Each constituency has been split into two to create two neighbourhoods with as equal sized population as possible.

Each neighbourhood is thus represented by a half hexagon. Each hexagon representing a constituency has been split into its two constituent neighbourhoods as they are related to each other in real space. So, for example Aberavon West lies to the left of Aberavon East, and Kirkcaldy South lies below Kirkcaldy North in the maps.

Figure 1 shows the regions and countries of Great Britain on the hexagonal cartogram and also on a conventional area map. To make reading of the maps easier we have separated the regions out slightly and marked out the lower course of the River Thames. Notice the difference in the size of London on the two maps.

Figure 2 shows the location of some cities and towns on both the cartogram and the conventional map to aid navigation. The outer boundary of Outer London coincides with the London region boundary. On all of the maps in this atlas the outlines of these urban areas are shown. Notice how all the cities and towns are much larger on the cartogram than on the conventional map. The size of every area is in proportion to its population. The locational appendix at the back of this atlas has a numbered map of all the neighbourhoods and a table of all the neighbourhoods with their numbers and names. Detailed, labelled cartograms of regions, countries and their constituent constituencies and neighbourhoods, together with a look-up table and an explanation of how to find a location given a name, and a name given a location, can be found on the accompanying website at (https://www.policypress.org.uk/page.php?name=9781861348241). Space limits precluded the inclusion of these maps in this atlas.

Figure 1: Regions and countries of Britain

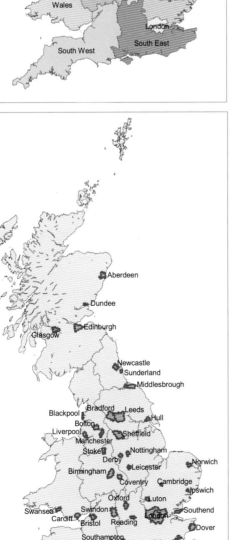

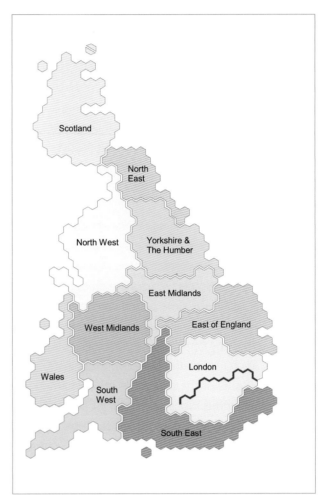

Figure 2: Selected towns and cities

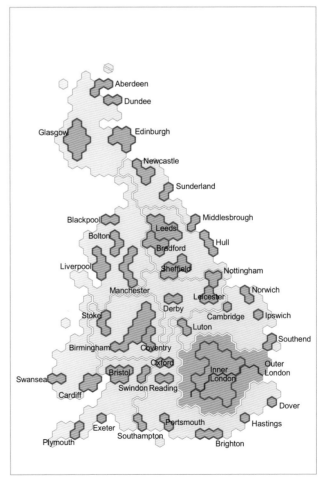

3 Technical notes

This section presents brief technical notes of how we created this atlas. Detailed explanations can be found in the Technical Appendix at the end of this atlas. Included there is an explanation of the Standardised Mortality Ratio (SMR), the number we calculate to show the incidence of a category of death, which takes into account the size and age and sex distribution of the population to show how much rates are above or below the average. The average, or national SMR, is always 100.

Throughout this atlas, for ease of comparison, we have used the same colouring scale for all the maps of incidence. This does not mean that every map and shade of colour on each map is strictly comparable, or that every shade of colour carries equal weight. One disadvantage of using the same colouring scheme throughout the atlas is that we have to show as much detail for rare causes of death – where chance influences the patterns shown far more – as we show for common causes of death (where the chances have been evened out by the weight of numbers). Readers should be particularly cautious of drawing implications from particular shades when the map as a whole is based on less than 5,000 deaths: an average of less than five deaths in each neighbourhood. This is because a single death can alter the ratio shown for a particular neighbourhood. You will see that a rare cause of death frequently results in a much wider range of SMRs, with sizeable numbers of places with an SMR of 400 and above, and others of below 25. In the key to each map we omit colours in the scale that do not appear on the map, so that the number of colours left indicates the range of possible scores. Choosing to sum all the deaths from a 24-year period has reduced the problems introduced by small numbers of deaths, but not eliminated them entirely.

The maps are based on the home addresses of the dead given on the death certificate. This means, for instance, that when a noticeable number of deaths occur from an accident, it will only show up on the maps if the people involved lived locally. Deaths associated with holiday and sporting activities, and traffic accidents, affect the death rates of the places where the people come from, not necessarily of where the death occurred. Similarly, many people die when they are in a hospital bed, but their death is recorded as if they died in their own home for the purposes of this mapping. So too for those who die in prison, but not for those usual residents of Britain who die overseas whose deaths cannot be included here. Princess Diana's death, for example, is not included in the map of motor vehicle accident deaths. The long-term residents of nursing homes and hospices, who have lived at their current address for more than six months, are usually shown here by their nursing home or hospice address. The precise rules that apply have changed over time and we give details in the Technical Appendix.

Some 14,833,696 death records were used in drawing up these maps. When people usually resident abroad die in Britain their death record contains no British address. Deaths with no such geography (35,818 cases or 0.24%) have been excluded, as have deaths with a geography but no cause of death code (a further 38,301 cases or 0.26%). Deaths with no geography are almost all deaths of visitors to the UK. A small but important number are bodies of homeless people found and not identified. Almost all of these bodies were found in London over the course of these years. Deaths with no cause of death code were not included, as in the raw data, some years had a range of ages and some years had all ages reported as zero.

4 What are you most likely to die of, when and where?

Different causes of death are more common at different ages and the risks vary by sex. Figure 3 shows the combination bar chart of groups of death nationally for each age band, divided into male and female. The age bands are of infants aged under 1, children aged 1-4, and then by five-year age bands, with the oldest group being people in their 90s and over. The bar charts are ordered so that the causes with most deaths are at the centre. The outer sections are all other causes of death for that age/sex group. This figure shows that for those who die in their first year of life, the large majority of fatalities are recorded as being due to none of the eight groups of causes shown. By the age of 40 the majority of deaths are from cardiovascular diseases or cancers and this is the case right up to age 90 when other causes again grow in importance. Between ages 5 and 35 a large, often the largest, cause of death is transport related, most commonly road traffic accidents.

Figure 4 displays the data for the exact same national distribution as measured over 24 years but here with individual causes of death identified rather than groups. When this is done the major causes of death for infants are made clear. As many individual causes of death as we could show on a graph, including all the major causes for infants and children as well as adults, are included here.

Figure 3: Age–sex bar chart by combined groups of cause of death, 1981–2004

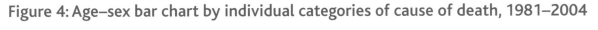

Legend:
- All cardiovascular deaths
- All cancer deaths
- All respiratory deaths
- All suicide/undetermined deaths
- All mental disorder deaths
- All transport deaths
- All deaths due to infections
- All homicide
- Other causes

Age axis (top to bottom): 90+, 85–89, 80–84, 75–79, 70–74, 65–69, 60–64, 55–59, 50–54, 45–49, 40–44, 35–39, 30–34, 25–29, 20–24, 15–19, 10–14, 5–9, 1–4, 0

Percent axis: 100 75 50 25 0 25 50 75 100
Males — Percent — Females

Note: the same colours are used as on the maps depicting the most common groups at each age band.

Figure 4: Age–sex bar chart by individual categories of cause of death, 1981–2004

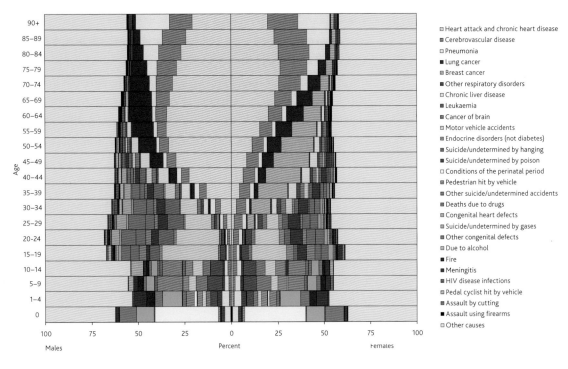

Legend:
- Heart attack and chronic heart disease
- Cerebrovascular disease
- Pneumonia
- Lung cancer
- Breast cancer
- Other respiratory disorders
- Chronic liver disease
- Leukaemia
- Cancer of brain
- Motor vehicle accidents
- Endocrine disorders (not diabetes)
- Suicide/undetermined by hanging
- Suicide/undetermined by poison
- Conditions of the perinatal period
- Pedestrian hit by vehicle
- Other suicide/undetermined accidents
- Deaths due to drugs
- Congenital heart defects
- Suicide/undetermined by gases
- Other congenital defects
- Due to alcohol
- Fire
- Meningitis
- HIV disease infections
- Pedal cyclist hit by vehicle
- Assault by cutting
- Assault using firearms
- Other causes

Age axis (top to bottom): 90+, 85–89, 80–84, 75–79, 70–74, 65–69, 60–64, 55–59, 50–54, 45–49, 40–44, 35–39, 30–34, 25–29, 20-24, 15–19, 10–14, 5–9, 1–4, 0

Percent axis: 100 75 50 25 0 25 50 75 100
Males — Percent — Females

Note: the same colours are used as on the maps depicting the most common cause of death at each age band.

Figure 5: Age–sex bar chart by most common causes of death for categories totalling more than 120,000 deaths nationally for the period 1981–2004

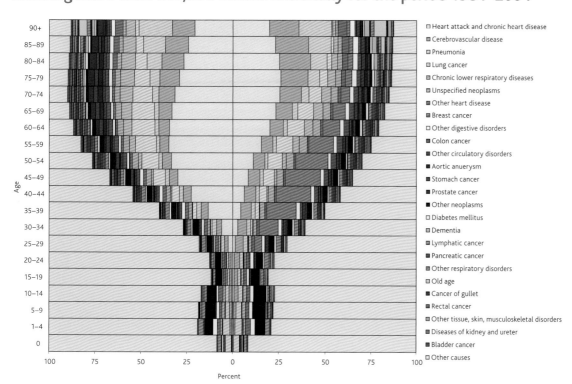

Finally in this series, Figure 5 shows the top causes of death by individual categories where there were over 120,000 deaths. Although this seems a rational selection, much of the important and interesting information about deaths of children and young adults is now absent.

Table 1 and Table 2 show the most common and second most common cause and group of deaths for each age band. These tables are for males and females combined. Separate tables for males and females are included in the Technical Appendix and show some significant differences at particular ages. Which causes are most common depends on how causes are grouped, how ages are grouped, what time period is being considered and the geographical extent of coverage. To recap, here the time period is 1981 to 2004 and the coverage is all of Britain. Table 1 shows that when you compare the 99 individual categories mapped in this atlas, five are the most common depending on age. A further seven entirely different categories are the second most common.

Decisions as to what categories to have and what to separate out can give a different slant to these figures, as shown in Table 2. Deaths involving transport, almost always involving cars, remain the most common cause of death between the ages of 10 and 24. Cardiovascular diseases are still the biggest killer over age 60. However, when all cancers are grouped, then as a group they are responsible for the majority of all deaths between the ages of 1–9 and 30–59. When all suicides are combined, they are the most important cause of death of people in their late twenties. Added to the suicide death count are others, most of which are likely to have been suicides, but where no evidence that the person intended to commit suicide was found. Similarly, combined respiratory diseases, when aggregated, are the major cause of death in infancy.

For each of the cause maps which follow in this atlas we present the average age of death from that cause. However, these individual cause maps give no indication of the major causes of death for each age group, so to give some context we have mapped here the most common cause of death for infants under 1, children aged 1 to 4, and then by five-year age bands with the final age group being people in their 90s and over. Where two causes are equally common in a particular place, we have chosen to map the one that has the younger average age of death.

Table 1: Most common and second most common causes of death at each age band out of 99 categories

Age	Most common cause of death	Second most common cause of death
0	Conditions of the perinatal period	Sudden death, cause unknown
1–4	Congenital heart defects	Other nervous disorders
5–9	Pedestrian hit by vehicle	Other nervous disorders
10–14	Pedestrian hit by vehicle	Other nervous disorders
15–19	Motor vehicle accidents	Other nervous disorders
20–24	Motor vehicle accidents	Deaths due to drugs
25–29	Motor vehicle accidents	Deaths due to drugs
30–34	Motor vehicle accidents	Deaths due to drugs
35–39	Heart attack and chronic heart disease	Breast cancer
40–44	Heart attack and chronic heart disease	Breast cancer
45–49	Heart attack and chronic heart disease	Breast cancer
50–54	Heart attack and chronic heart disease	Lung cancer
55–59	Heart attack and chronic heart disease	Lung cancer
60–64	Heart attack and chronic heart disease	Lung cancer
65–69	Heart attack and chronic heart disease	Lung cancer
70–74	Heart attack and chronic heart disease	Cerebrovascular disease
75-79	Heart attack and chronic heart disease	Cerebrovascular disease
80–84	Heart attack and chronic heart disease	Cerebrovascular disease
85–89	Heart attack and chronic heart disease	Cerebrovascular disease
90+	Heart attack and chronic heart disease	Pneumonia

Table 2: Most common and second most common causes of death at each age band out of 9 groups

Age	Most common group of death	Second most common group of death
0	All respiratory deaths	All deaths due to infections
1–4	All cancer deaths	All respiratory deaths
5–9	All cancer deaths	All transport deaths
10–14	All transport deaths	All cancer deaths
15–19	All transport deaths	All suicide/undetermined deaths
20–24	All transport deaths	All suicide/undetermined deaths
25–29	All suicide/undetermined deaths	All cancer deaths
30–34	All cancer deaths	All suicide/undetermined deaths
35–39	All cancer deaths	All cardiovascular deaths
40–44	All cancer deaths	All cardiovascular deaths
45–49	All cancer deaths	All cardiovascular deaths
50–54	All cancer deaths	All cardiovascular deaths
55–59	All cancer deaths	All cardiovascular deaths
60–64	All cardiovascular deaths	All cancer deaths
65–69	All cardiovascular deaths	All cancer deaths
70–74	All cardiovascular deaths	All cancer deaths
75–79	All cardiovascular deaths	All cancer deaths
80–84	All cardiovascular deaths	All cancer deaths
85–89	All cardiovascular deaths	All respiratory deaths
90+	All cardiovascular deaths	All respiratory deaths

Group maps

We have mapped the group of deaths that is the most common cause of death for each age band. The groups are of selected causes of death – cardiovascular, cancer, respiratory, infections, mental disorder, transport, suicide or undetermined, and homicide. For the groups, we have suppressed data for those neighbourhoods where there were very few deaths for any particular age band there. In this series of maps, each group is depicted by the same colour, but colours not appearing on a map are omitted from its legend.

Of the deaths that occur in infancy (age 0), in the groups, the most common cause of death is respiratory. Note that where there were very small numbers of deaths we have suppressed the data.

Between the ages of 1 and 4, there is a much wider variety of causes of death groups, but little geographical patterning apart from transport being more prevalent as a cause of death in the northern part of the country than the south.

For the next age group, 5–9, transport deaths dominate the northern half of the map even more, while childhood cancers are the most common causes of death in the southern parts of the country.

By the ages of 10 to 14, deaths from traffic are most common across even more of the country.

As we move on to the next age band, 15–19, the shades on the map change radically. In most places, the most common cause of death for older teenagers is transport. In comparison, in many urban areas, the prevailing cause of death is suicide or undetermined intent. Two neighbourhoods in Glasgow have homicide as the most common cause of death for this age group.

By the early twenties (20–24), transport and suicide or undetermined remain the most common groups but suicide or undetermined intent is much more prevalent, with almost all of the urban areas having this as the most common cause of death. The Easterhouse neighbourhood of Glasgow is the only place where homicide was the leading cause of death in this period. Homicide does not appear on any of the older age group maps, but appears somewhere on every map for every younger age group.

As we move into the late twenties (25–29), deaths due to transport are the most common cause in a decreasing number of places. Suicides and undetermined intent are the most common cause of death at these ages across much of the country, while we start to see cancer as the leading cause of death in a scattering of places.

At ages 30–34 the map colours change radically again, with cancer the dominant colour on the map, particularly in rural areas. Suicide and undetermined intent remain the most common cause in many urban areas, transport remains the most common killer in a few more rural places and we start to see cardiovascular causes appearing.

By the ages of 35–39 the map is dominated by cancer as the most common cause of death, with cardiovascular causes particularly evident in northern urban areas as an early determinant of premature mortality before age 40.

There then follows a series of maps covering the five-year age bands from 40–44 through to 70–74. On all of these maps the most common causes of death are cardiovascular or cancer and they show the changing geographical variation across these years of age. At younger ages cardiovascular causes dominate in the northern parts of the country and London, and gradually extend southwards and eastwards. By ages 65–69, cardiovascular is the most common cause of death across almost all of the country, apart from a ring in the south east around London where cancer dominates. At 70–74, only one neighbourhood, Surrey Heath North, has cancer as the most common cause of death, the rest of Britain having cardiovascular as the main cause.

At ages 75 and over, the leading cause of death in every neighbourhood is cardiovascular and so the whole map is a single colour.

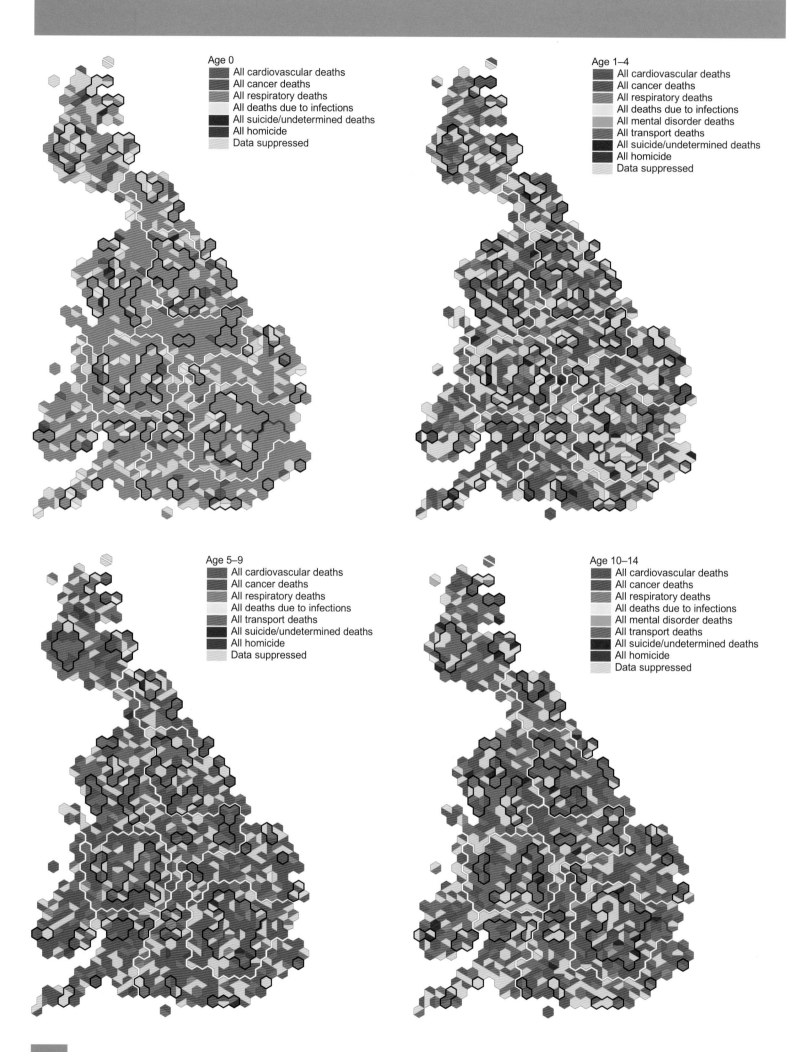

Age 0
- All cardiovascular deaths
- All cancer deaths
- All respiratory deaths
- All deaths due to infections
- All suicide/undetermined deaths
- All homicide
- Data suppressed

Age 1–4
- All cardiovascular deaths
- All cancer deaths
- All respiratory deaths
- All deaths due to infections
- All mental disorder deaths
- All transport deaths
- All suicide/undetermined deaths
- All homicide
- Data suppressed

Age 5–9
- All cardiovascular deaths
- All cancer deaths
- All respiratory deaths
- All deaths due to infections
- All transport deaths
- All suicide/undetermined deaths
- All homicide
- Data suppressed

Age 10–14
- All cardiovascular deaths
- All cancer deaths
- All respiratory deaths
- All deaths due to infections
- All mental disorder deaths
- All transport deaths
- All suicide/undetermined deaths
- All homicide
- Data suppressed

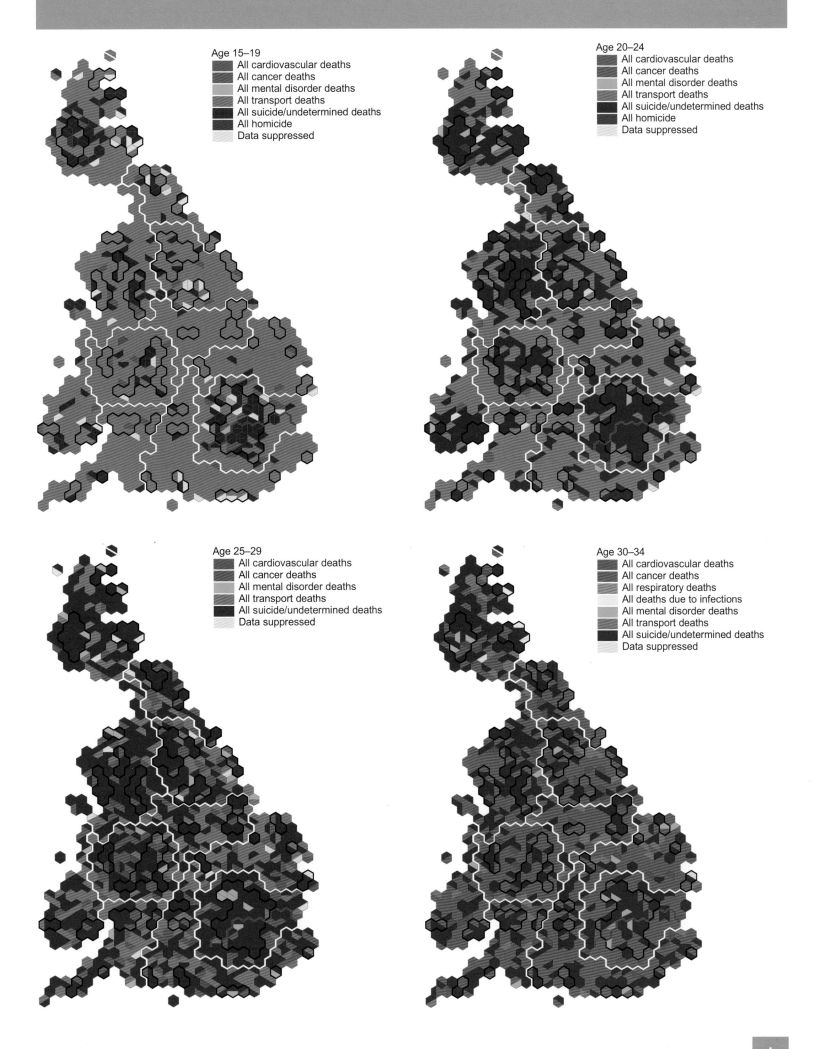

Age 15–19
- All cardiovascular deaths
- All cancer deaths
- All mental disorder deaths
- All transport deaths
- All suicide/undetermined deaths
- All homicide
- Data suppressed

Age 20–24
- All cardiovascular deaths
- All cancer deaths
- All mental disorder deaths
- All transport deaths
- All suicide/undetermined deaths
- All homicide
- Data suppressed

Age 25–29
- All cardiovascular deaths
- All cancer deaths
- All mental disorder deaths
- All transport deaths
- All suicide/undetermined deaths
- Data suppressed

Age 30–34
- All cardiovascular deaths
- All cancer deaths
- All respiratory deaths
- All deaths due to infections
- All mental disorder deaths
- All transport deaths
- All suicide/undetermined deaths
- Data suppressed

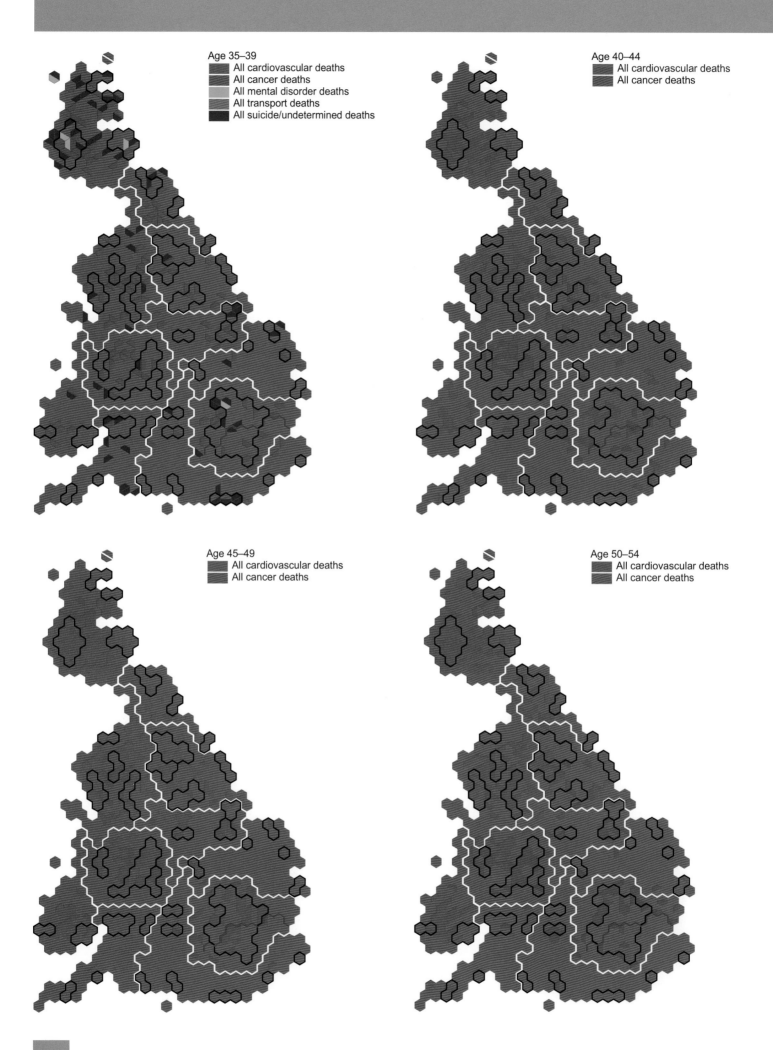

Age 35–39
- All cardiovascular deaths
- All cancer deaths
- All mental disorder deaths
- All transport deaths
- All suicide/undetermined deaths

Age 40–44
- All cardiovascular deaths
- All cancer deaths

Age 45–49
- All cardiovascular deaths
- All cancer deaths

Age 50–54
- All cardiovascular deaths
- All cancer deaths

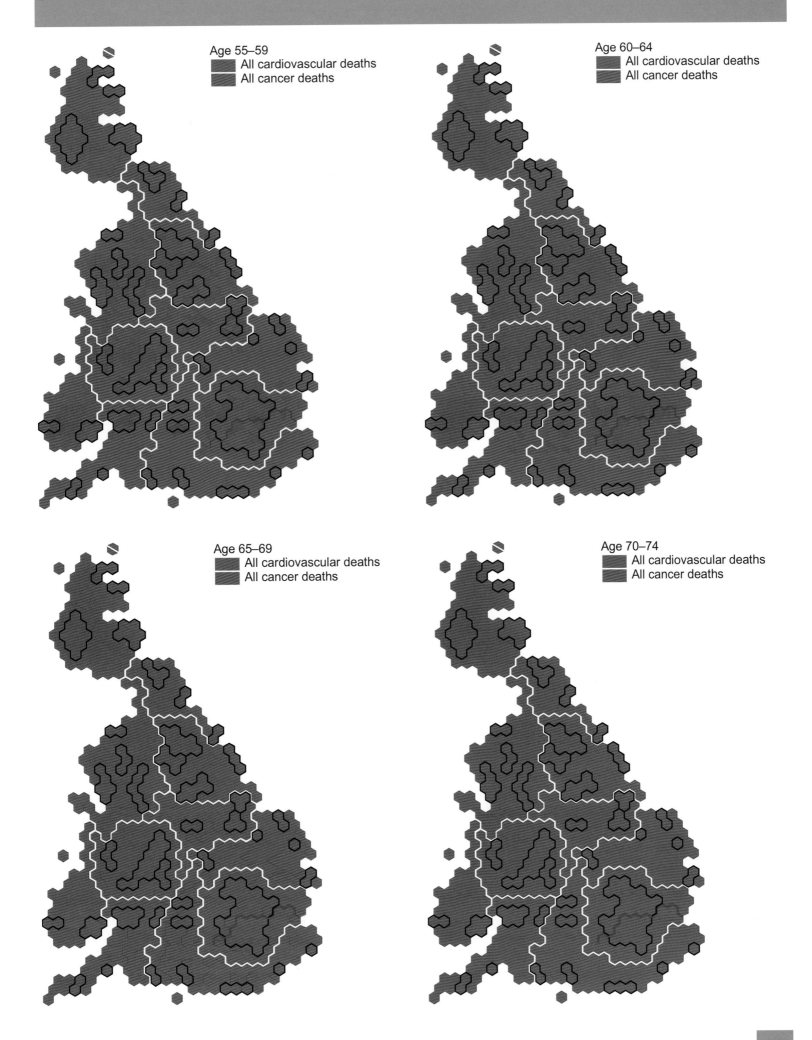

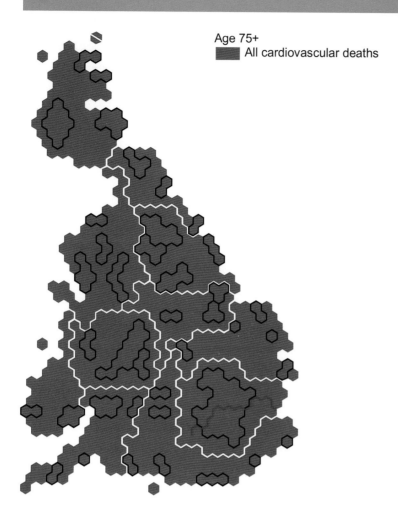

Age 75+

All cardiovascular deaths

Single category maps

The next series of maps are of the most common *single* category of death. 26 of our 99 categories are shown by the same 26 separate colours. When a neighbourhood's most common cause of death for that age group is not included in those colours it is shown as an *Other cause* category. Colours that do not appear on a particular map are not shown in its legend.

For infants aged 0, the most common cause of death across most of the country is *Conditions of the perinatal period*. Of those neighbourhoods where this is not the case, most fall into the *Other cause* category. There are five neighbourhoods with another identified cause: *Congenital heart defects* in Ellesmere Port West, *Other congenital defects* in Hexham West, Keighley North and Meirionnydd Urban, and *Other respiratory disorders* in Nottingham Bilborough. The categories referred to as 'Other' refer to certain deaths from that cause having been excluded. The main maps give full explanations of each category.

Very few young children die after reaching their first birthday; when they do die it is often not from any common cause. On the map of the most common cause of death at ages 1–4 much

of the country is categorised as *Other cause*. The greens of *Congenital defects* are the most common cause in many places, with a clear preponderance of deaths due to fire in Scotland.

At ages 5–9, we again find that much of the country is categorised as *Other cause*. Here we see the oranges of road traffic accidents predominating across much of the country, with *Pedestrian hit by vehicle* more prevalent across the northern part of Britain. We would not normally expect to see *Assault using firearms* as the major cause of death of children of these ages: the two such neighbourhoods in Scotland are where the children who were killed in the Dunblane massacre lived.

By ages 10–14, where it is not *Other cause* that is the predominant category, we again find road traffic accidents predominating in many parts of the country. The prevalence of road traffic accidents continues through the years of young adulthood. At ages 15–19, *Motor vehicle accidents* are the leading cause of death across most of the country, with *Suicide/undetermined accidents* dominating London and parts of Scotland and *Deaths due to drugs* dominating much of urban Scotland.

By the early twenties (20–24), *Suicide/undetermined accidents* and *Deaths due to drugs* are the majority killers across much of urban Britain; by the latter half of this decade of life (25–29), these two causes have spread into more rural areas, but *Motor vehicle accidents* remain the leading cause of death across most of rural Britain. These are accidents resulting in the deaths of drivers and/or passengers.

As we move into the next stage of life, in many places external causes of death start to be overtaken by what are often seen as more natural causes (diseases). The map of the major cause of death at ages 30–34 is essentially that of those 5 years younger, but with some places where heart attacks and cancers have become the leading cause of death. Dundee, Edinburgh, Scunthorpe North, and the Queensbury, West Norwood, Blackheath, Bermondsey and Tottenham neighbourhoods of London all have *HIV disease infections* as the leading cause of death. In some cases this is because of where particular medical facilities were located in the past.

By the late thirties (35–39), suicides and road traffic accidents are no longer the leading cause of death in so many places. The pale pink of *Heart attack and chronic heart disease* dominates much of the map, particularly in the north, while in the south breast cancer is the leading killer. In Scotland deaths *Due to alcohol* and *Chronic liver disease* start to dominate, while Inner London has a preponderance of neighbourhoods where *Pneumonia* predominates. In the early years of the period being mapped here, young people who would later have been said to have died of *HIV disease infections* often had the cause recorded as *Pneumonia*.

The next map, of the major cause of death at ages 40–44, is a much simpler map. *Heart attack and chronic heart disease* is the majority killer almost everywhere, and where it is not, *Breast cancer* is the leading cause of death, prevalent in more southern neighbourhoods than northern.

By the late 40s (45–49), only three causes of death are in the majority in any place: *Heart attack and chronic heart disease, Breast cancer* and *Lung cancer*. The latter is found in only one neighbourhood, Llandudno in north Wales. Again, a particularly rare cluster such as this is quite likely to have been associated with a place and time when people suffering from this disease may have gone to convalesce.

In the age group 50–54, virtually the entire country has *Heart attack and chronic heart disease* as the leading cause of death. The one exception is the neighbourhood of Great Shelford in Cambridgeshire where the leading cause over these 24 years was *Breast cancer*.

Heart attack and chronic heart disease is the leading cause of death for every neighbourhood for the following six five-year age bands, from 55 to 84, so are all mapped together on one single map.

It is not until we reach the 85–89 age band that we again start to see any variation in the leading cause of death. *Heart attack and chronic heart disease* still predominate, but there are a handful of neighbourhoods where *Cerebrovascular disease* or *Pneumonia* predominate.

Finally, for those aged 90 and over, the leading causes of death are *Heart attack and chronic heart disease* and *Pneumonia* across most of the country, with *Cerebrovascular disease* more prevalent in Scotland.

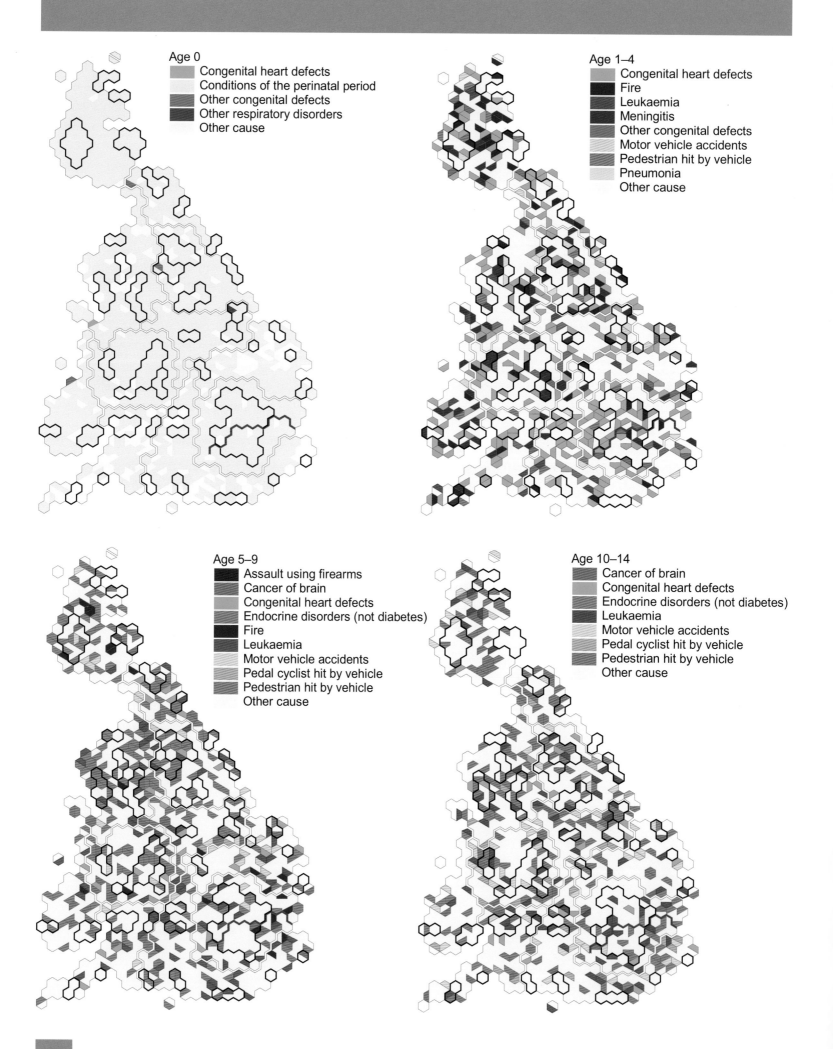

Age 0
- Congenital heart defects
- Conditions of the perinatal period
- Other congenital defects
- Other respiratory disorders
- Other cause

Age 1–4
- Congenital heart defects
- Fire
- Leukaemia
- Meningitis
- Other congenital defects
- Motor vehicle accidents
- Pedestrian hit by vehicle
- Pneumonia
- Other cause

Age 5–9
- Assault using firearms
- Cancer of brain
- Congenital heart defects
- Endocrine disorders (not diabetes)
- Fire
- Leukaemia
- Motor vehicle accidents
- Pedal cyclist hit by vehicle
- Pedestrian hit by vehicle
- Other cause

Age 10–14
- Cancer of brain
- Congenital heart defects
- Endocrine disorders (not diabetes)
- Leukaemia
- Motor vehicle accidents
- Pedal cyclist hit by vehicle
- Pedestrian hit by vehicle
- Other cause

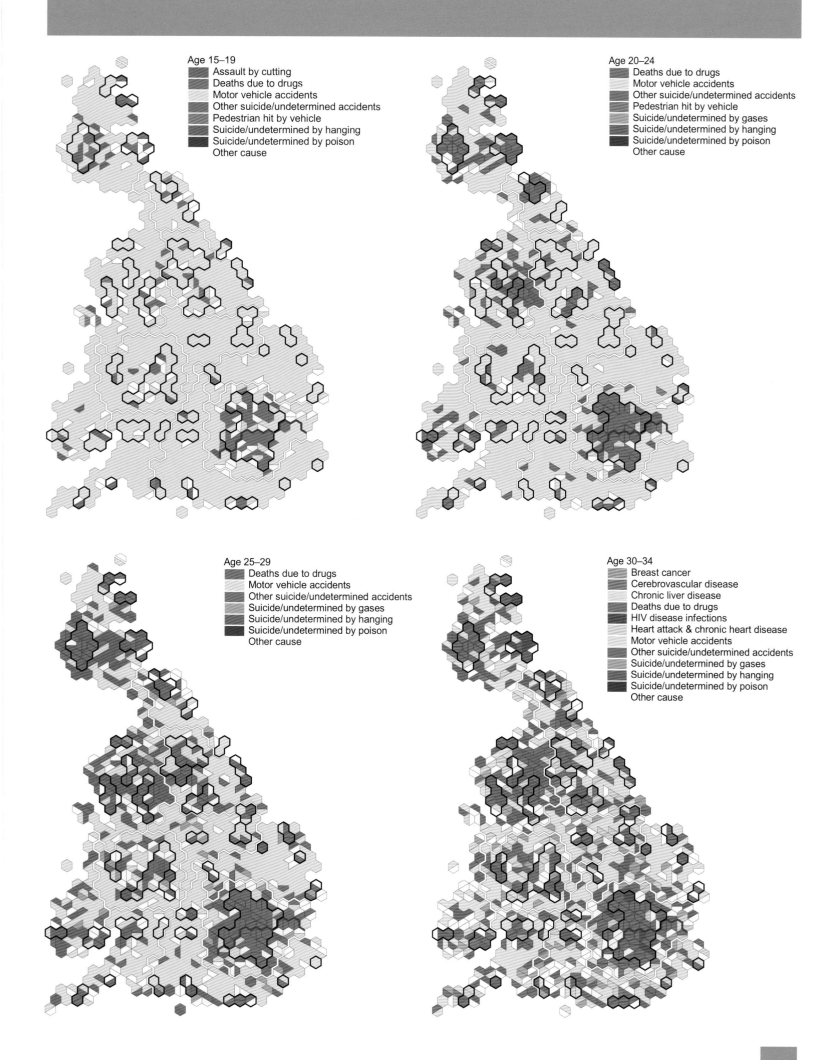

Age 15–19
- Assault by cutting
- Deaths due to drugs
- Motor vehicle accidents
- Other suicide/undetermined accidents
- Pedestrian hit by vehicle
- Suicide/undetermined by hanging
- Suicide/undetermined by poison
- Other cause

Age 20–24
- Deaths due to drugs
- Motor vehicle accidents
- Other suicide/undetermined accidents
- Pedestrian hit by vehicle
- Suicide/undetermined by gases
- Suicide/undetermined by hanging
- Suicide/undetermined by poison
- Other cause

Age 25–29
- Deaths due to drugs
- Motor vehicle accidents
- Other suicide/undetermined accidents
- Suicide/undetermined by gases
- Suicide/undetermined by hanging
- Suicide/undetermined by poison
- Other cause

Age 30–34
- Breast cancer
- Cerebrovascular disease
- Chronic liver disease
- Deaths due to drugs
- HIV disease infections
- Heart attack & chronic heart disease
- Motor vehicle accidents
- Other suicide/undetermined accidents
- Suicide/undetermined by gases
- Suicide/undetermined by hanging
- Suicide/undetermined by poison
- Other cause

| Years of life lost (million years) | | Death before age 75 | | | % of years | Cumulative |
Map	Cause	Males	Females	People	lost	percentage
Map 28	HIV disease infections	0.21	0.05	0.25	0.294	96
Map 27	Accidental drowning	0.21	0.05	0.25	0.293	96
Map 73	Septicaemia	0.12	0.10	0.23	0.263	96
Map 76	Other uterine cancer	0.00	0.21	0.21	0.249	97
Map 51	Ill-defined and unknown causes	0.14	0.06	0.20	0.237	97
Map 45	Choking on food	0.12	0.07	0.19	0.217	97
Map 33	Suicide/undetermined by jumping	0.13	0.05	0.18	0.210	97
Map 25	Pedal cyclist hit by vehicle	0.15	0.03	0.18	0.208	97
Map 63	Bronchitis	0.10	0.08	0.18	0.204	98
Map 65	Laryngeal cancer	0.14	0.03	0.17	0.193	98
Map 21	Other assaults	0.10	0.07	0.17	0.193	98
Map 35	Suicide/undetermined by firearms	0.13	0.01	0.13	0.156	98
Map 103	Other genitourinary disorders	0.06	0.07	0.13	0.146	98
Map 66	Tuberculosis infections	0.08	0.05	0.12	0.144	98
Map 107	Other mental disorders	0.06	0.06	0.12	0.141	99
Map 18	Assault by cutting	0.08	0.02	0.11	0.124	99
Map 36	Other accidental poisoning	0.08	0.02	0.10	0.116	99
Map 94	Industrial lung diseases	0.07	0.03	0.10	0.115	99
Map 106	Dementia	0.05	0.05	0.10	0.112	99
Map 101	Parkinson's disease	0.06	0.03	0.09	0.109	99
Map 69	During surgery, medical care	0.04	0.03	0.07	0.082	99
Map 108	Atherosclerosis	0.04	0.02	0.07	0.078	99
Map 39	Suicide/undetermined by cutting	0.05	0.01	0.07	0.076	99
Map 26	Railway accidents	0.06	0.01	0.06	0.073	99
Map 44	Hepatitis	0.04	0.02	0.06	0.071	100
Map 30	Caused by machinery	0.06	0.00	0.06	0.068	100
Map 17	Accidental deaths due to electric current	0.05	0.01	0.06	0.064	100
Map 16	Pregnancy and childbirth	0.00	0.05	0.05	0.063	100
Map 24	Water transport accidents	0.04	0.00	0.04	0.045	100
Map 102	Influenza	0.02	0.02	0.04	0.041	100
Map 81	Hypothermia	0.02	0.01	0.03	0.038	100
Map 29	Air accidents	0.03	0.00	0.03	0.037	100
Map 20	Assault using firearms	0.02	0.01	0.03	0.035	100
Map 80	Signs and symptoms	0.02	0.01	0.03	0.032	100
Map 50	Hunger, thirst, exposure, neglect	0.01	0.01	0.02	0.021	100
Map 104	Other intestinal infections	0.01	0.01	0.01	0.016	100
Map 109	Old age	0.00	0.00	0.00	0.003	100

Table 4: Years of life lost for 10 grouped causes of death, 1981–2004

| Years of life lost (million years) | | Death before age 75 | | | % of years lost |
Map	Grouping	Males	Females	People	
Map 1	All deaths	53.11	32.90	86.01	100.00
Map 2	All homicide	0.20	0.10	0.30	0.35
Map 3	All transport deaths	2.75	0.77	3.52	4.09
Map 4	All suicide/undetermined deaths	3.49	1.15	4.64	5.40
Map 5	All external deaths	8.16	2.64	10.80	12.56
Map 6	All deaths due to infections	0.69	0.38	1.07	1.25
Map 7	All cancer deaths	13.57	12.75	26.32	30.60
Map 8	All mental disorder deaths	1.17	0.41	1.58	1.84
Map 9	All cardiovascular deaths	17.27	7.73	25.00	29.06
Map 10	All respiratory deaths	3.43	2.30	5.73	6.66

Note: the groupings are not exhaustive and so do not sum to all deaths. Therefore, no cumulative percentage is given.

6 How to use this atlas

These two pages explain the layout of the main body of the atlas and describe the various parts of each page.

Map number and title

Number of deaths from this cause

Proportion of all deaths that this cause accounts for

18 ASSAULT BY CUTTING

2,645 cases

0.02% of all deaths

average age = 34.8

male:female ratio = 75:25

This cause of death comes under the 'external' causes of death category (see Map 5) and falls into the sub-category of 'Homicide and injury purposely inflicted by other persons', along with a range of other methods of murder/assault, such as use of firearms or poisoning. See also Map 39 Suicide/undetermined by cutting.

Details of the cause of death and to which category it belongs.

Also references to maps of similar causes.

The average age of death from this cause

Male to female ratio of deaths from this cause

Three quarters of those who have died due to this cause are males. As the age–sex bar chart shows, younger males are at a much higher risk. The rates in Glasgow and the south west of Scotland are immediately striking. London and other English urban centres follow with the next highest SMRs. Much of the remainder of rural and provincial Britain has substantially lower rates.

This cause of death includes killing by cutting or stabbing using a sharp object, most commonly a knife or broken glass. It includes killing which may be intentional or unintentional; many of these assaults are impulsive, related to alcohol and drug misuse, and assailants use whatever weapon is to hand. Often the knife used is a kitchen knife in a domestic incident. Women are more commonly murdered by their partners. Men are more commonly murdered by someone to whom they are unrelated.

A discussion of the cause of death is here, together with commentary on the map. There may also be a diagram or a photograph on this page.

Blunt-ended table knives were introduced in the 18th century to reduce the injuries resulting from arguments over the dinner table in public eateries (Hern et al, 2005). Many domestic kitchen knives, however, are of the dagger variety with a pointed tip and they often have a long blade. In contrast to a knife with a short blade these can penetrate deeply and can easily cause serious injury or death. Hern and colleagues argue that there is no culinary necessity for knives of this type and that banning them would drastically reduce their availability and therefore their use in personal attacks.

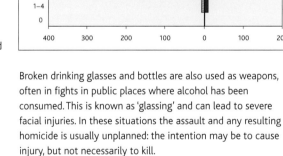

Some causes have an age–sex bar chart. This shows the number of deaths by sex, at age 0, age 1–4 and then by 5–year age band. We only show such charts where the age–sex distribution is particularly interesting

Broken drinking glasses and bottles are also used as weapons, often in fights in public places where alcohol has been consumed. This is known as 'glassing' and can lead to severe facial injuries. In these situations the assault and any resulting homicide is usually unplanned: the intention may be to cause injury, but not necessarily to kill.

Hern, E., Glazebrook, W. and Beckett, M. (2005) 'Reducing knife crime', *BMJ*, no 330, pp 1221-2.

Here we list all the ICD-9 and ICD-10 codes that make up this cause of death. See Technical Appendix.

ICD-9 codes: E966
ICD-10 codes: X99

ICD-9	ICD-9 name	% of cases	ICD-10	ICD-10 name	% of cases
E966	Assault by cutting and piercing instrument	100.0	X99	Assault by sharp object	100.0
		100.0			100.0

The table lists ICD codes and the percentage they comprise of the cause of death. If there are a large number of codes only those that make the largest contributon are shown, the remainder being grouped under 'other causes in group'

MAP 18   ASSAULT BY CUTTING

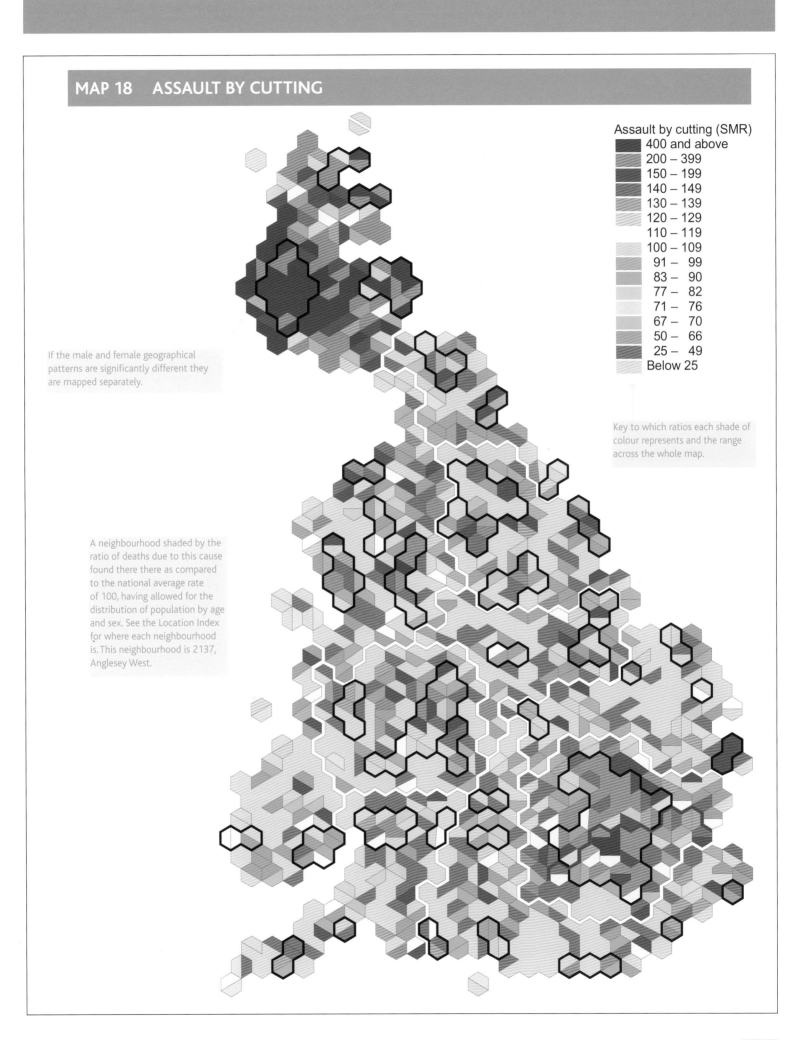

Assault by cutting (SMR)

- 400 and above
- 200 – 399
- 150 – 199
- 140 – 149
- 130 – 139
- 120 – 129
- 110 – 119
- 100 – 109
- 91 – 99
- 83 – 90
- 77 – 82
- 71 – 76
- 67 – 70
- 50 – 66
- 25 – 49
- Below 25

If the male and female geographical patterns are significantly different they are mapped separately.

Key to which ratios each shade of colour represents and the range across the whole map.

A neighbourhood shaded by the ratio of deaths due to this cause found there as compared to the national average rate of 100, having allowed for the distribution of population by age and sex. See the Location Index for where each neighbourhood is. This neighbourhood is 2137, Anglesey West.

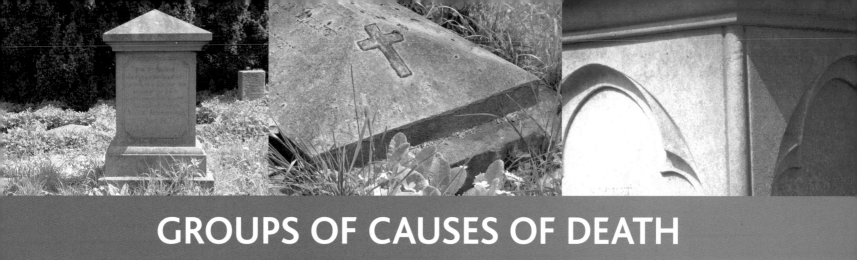

GROUPS OF CAUSES OF DEATH

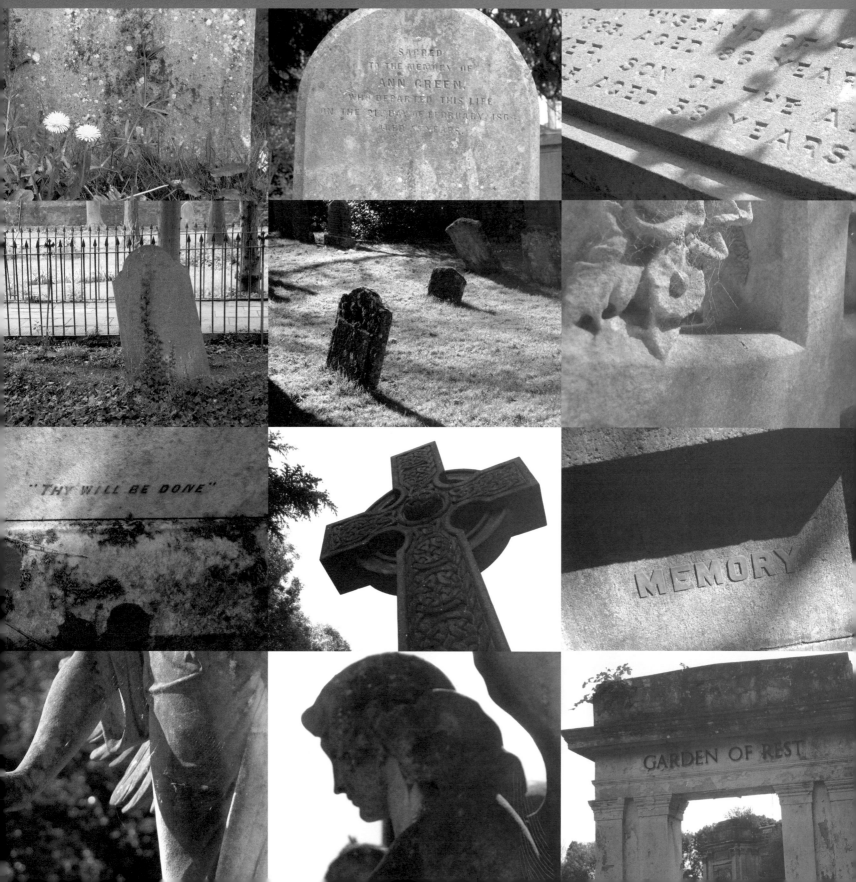

1   ALL DEATHS

This category includes *all* deaths in Britain (England, Scotland and Wales) between 1981 and 2004 inclusive.

14,833,696 cases

100% of all deaths

average age = 74.4

male:female ratio = 48:52

The map of mortality rates from all causes combines in a single image all the influences on our survival. Having taken into account the distribution of the population according to age and sex, the map shows that across these areas a person's chances of dying in a particular year varied from being more than 50% above the national average (an SMR of 150 as shown on the key) to less than 76% of the national average (with SMRs ranging from 71 to 76 in the lowest mortality category). Thus, depending on where you were living over the last quarter of a century, there are neighbourhoods of Britain containing populations of tens of thousands of people where you were more than twice as likely to die than had you lived in other places.

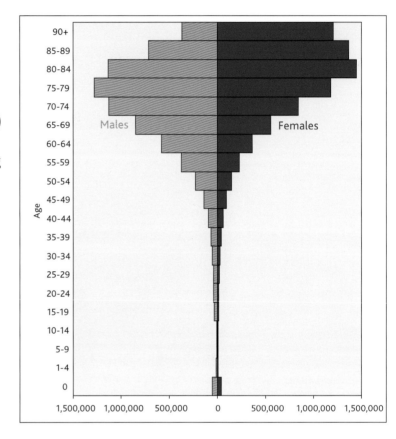

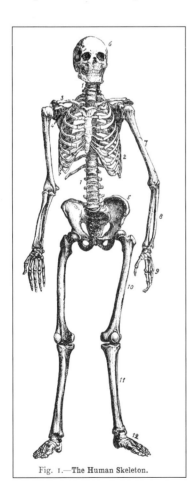

Fig. 1.—The Human Skeleton.

The 1,282 neighbourhoods shown here both physically and statistically collect groups of people together whose rates of dying vary considerably at the extremes. For the large majority in the middle, however, living in the areas with an SMR between 90 and 110, mortality rates do not appear to vary greatly. However, before concluding that this variation is low it is worth remembering that it is compound. If every year in certain towns in Britain an extra 10% of the population die than on average, whereas in another some 10% fewer die than you would expect given their ages and sexes, then the life expectancies of people in those two towns will diverge by several years.

Across much of the south of England outside London, and in a few isolated enclaves of prosperity in the north, Wales and Scotland, people's chances of dying each year have been at least 10%, often 20% and at the extremes almost 30% lower than average since 1981.

Over this 24-year period, the average age of death in Britain was 74.4 years, 71.2 for men and 77.4 for women. The average age of death in our neighbourhoods varied between 66.4 years (in Glasgow Easterhouse) and 80.6 years (in Eastbourne West). These are averages. The lower figures are due to many people dying much younger; the higher due to many people living longer. Over this period 42.0% of people who died were over 80 years old, while 12.4% were under 60 years old. In the worst neighbourhood 25.0% were under 60 years old.

MAP 1   ALL DEATHS

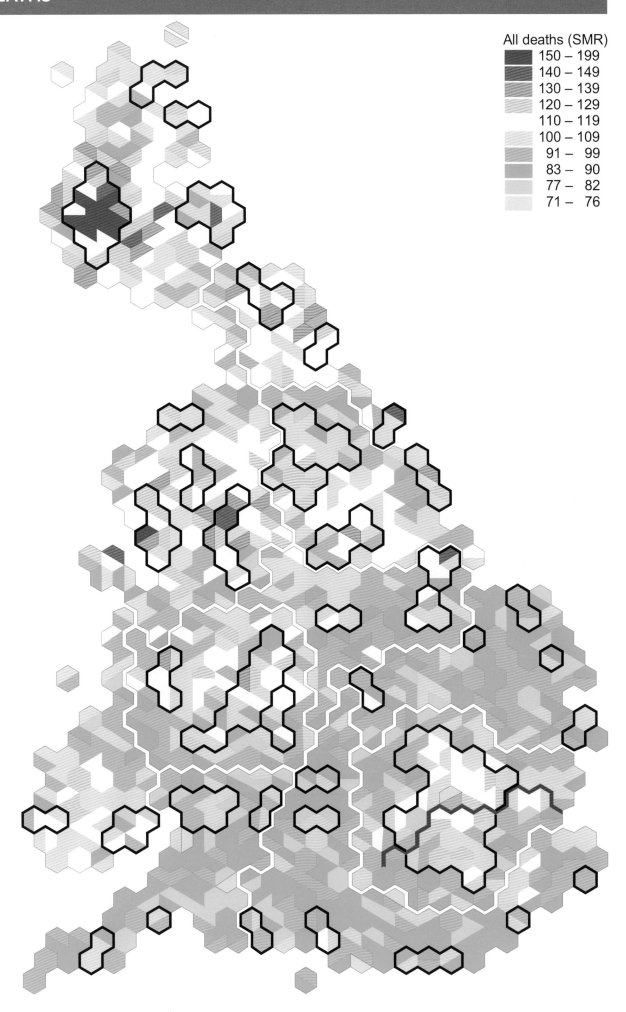

All deaths (SMR)

	150 – 199
	140 – 149
	130 – 139
	120 – 129
	110 – 119
	100 – 109
	91 – 99
	83 – 90
	77 – 82
	71 – 76

2 ALL HOMICIDE

This category includes all murders and is a sub-category of all external deaths (see Map 5).

7,677 cases

0.05% of all deaths

average age = 35.9

male:female ratio = 64:36

The map shows a concentration of higher murder rates in Scotland. Murder there, especially on the west coast, is more common than in the rest of Britain. It is only as common in the one part of Liverpool that also was the only area of England to have an overall mortality rate comparable to parts of Glasgow, and in one neighbourhood in south London. Across much of England, and even more of Wales, mortality rates from homicide are a quarter, half or three quarters of the national average rate and in several areas even lower than this.

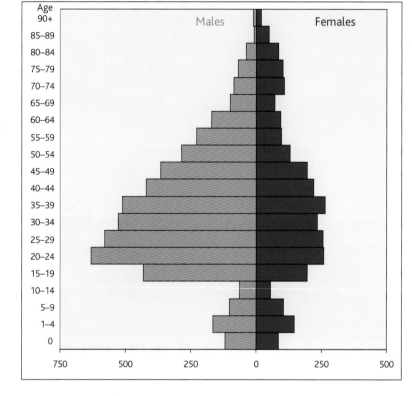

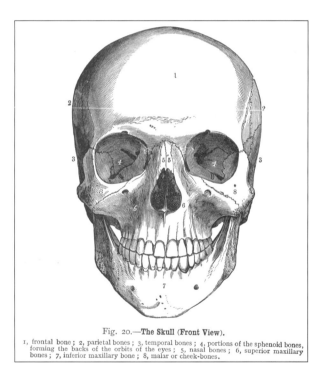

Fig. 20.—The Skull (Front View).

1, frontal bone ; 2, parietal bones ; 3, temporal bones ; 4, portions of the sphenoid bones, forming the backs of the orbits of the eyes ; 5, nasal bones ; 6, superior maxillary bones ; 7, inferior maxillary bone ; 8, malar or cheek-bones.

Group	Causes	Map	% of cases
All homicide	Assault by cutting	18	34.5
	Assault using firearms	20	9.8
	Other assaults	21	55.7
			100.0

The age–sex bar chart shows the age and sex distribution for those people whose deaths are recorded as murders. It shows that people of all ages are murdered, including young children. However, the total number of people murdered is relatively low, at an average of 320 a year or 6 per week; just one in 2,000 people die from this cause. Men are more likely to be victims of murder than are women, with rates being higher for men between the ages of 15 and 65. The average age of death of murder victims is just 35.9.

Deaths in England and Wales ascertained to be homicide more than a year after the event are not included in those mapped and counted here.

MAP 2A (FEMALES) 2B (MALES)   ALL HOMICIDE

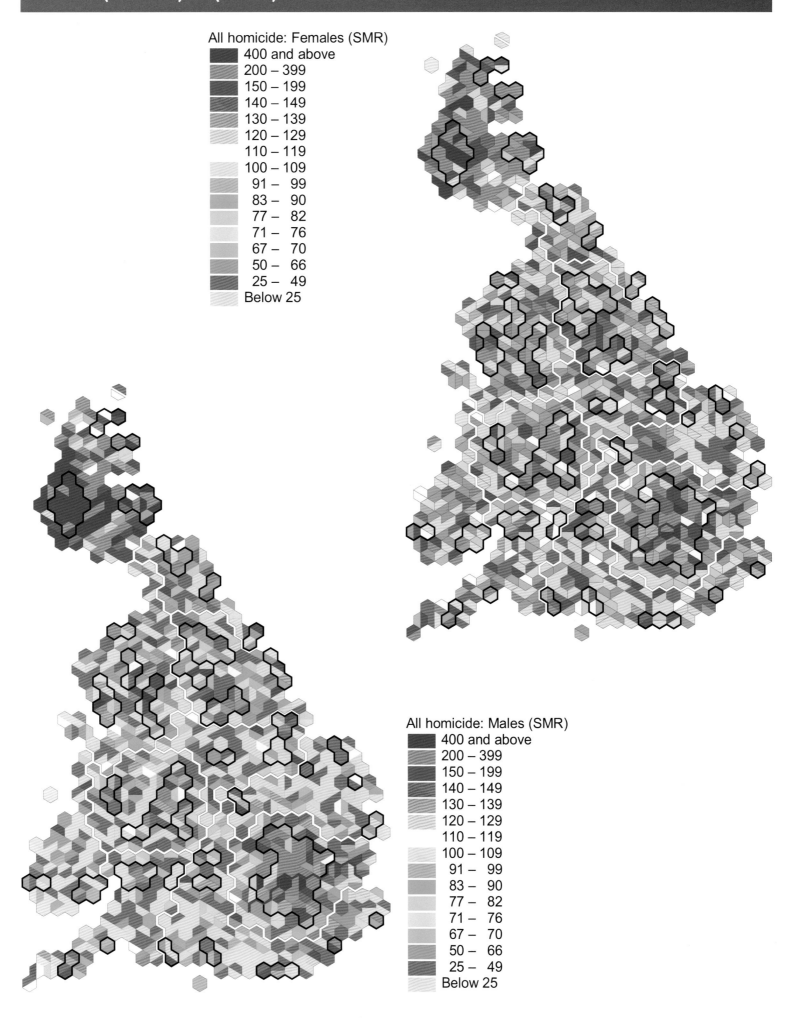

All homicide: Females (SMR)

	400 and above
	200 – 399
	150 – 199
	140 – 149
	130 – 139
	120 – 129
	110 – 119
	100 – 109
	91 – 99
	83 – 90
	77 – 82
	71 – 76
	67 – 70
	50 – 66
	25 – 49
	Below 25

All homicide: Males (SMR)

	400 and above
	200 – 399
	150 – 199
	140 – 149
	130 – 139
	120 – 129
	110 – 119
	100 – 109
	91 – 99
	83 – 90
	77 – 82
	71 – 76
	67 – 70
	50 – 66
	25 – 49
	Below 25

4   ALL SUICIDE/UNDETERMINED DEATHS

This is a sub-category of all external deaths (see Map 5) and includes suicides and deaths for which the intent remains undetermined as to whether it was suicide or an accident. It is likely that the majority of undetermined deaths were in fact suicides but there was insufficient evidence to establish that the intent was definitely suicide.

156,128 cases

1.05% of all deaths

average age = 45.8

male:female ratio = 71:29

Suicide rates tend to be higher in areas where people feel more isolated – in the centres of cities such as London, Brighton, Manchester and Glasgow, and in the remoter northern parts of Scotland. Rates are lowest in the more affluent parts of southern England where much higher than average proportions of people are in work and so are less isolated during the day, are better rewarded financially and are less likely to be single and as a result are less isolated outside of work. Furthermore, population turnover is lower so more people know their neighbours.

Outside of these general explanations of the geographical map of suicide, rates tend to be lower in areas where a higher proportion of people adhere to particular religions or denominations that view suicide as particularly transgressive.

Rates are also artificially elevated in Scotland because there the system of recording suicides initially labels more deaths as suicide than may be later found to actually be suicide, and it is an anomaly of this dataset that these deaths are not subsequently re-coded. To a small extent the inverse is the case in England and Wales where a coroner's inquest or court proceedings can take so long that a death is not registered as a suicide in time to be included in the data used here.

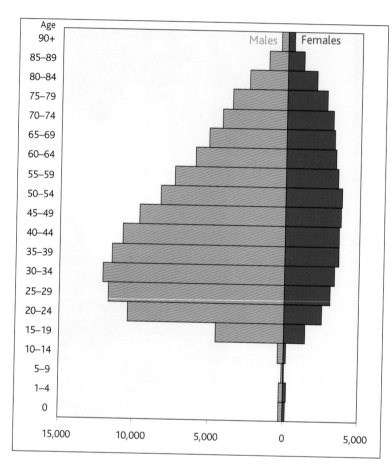

Group	Causes	Map	% of cases
All suicide/ undeter- mined deaths	Other suicide/undetermined accidents	31	17.5
	Suicide/undetermined by gases	32	13.5
	Suicide/undetermined by jumping	33	3.6
	Suicide/undetermined by hanging	34	26.8
	Suicide/undetermined by firearms	35	2.9
	Suicide/undetermined by poison	38	26.2
	Suicide/undetermined by cutting	39	1.7
	Suicide/undetermined by drowning	42	7.8
			100.0

The average age of death for this cause is 45.8 years. Seven out of ten of the deaths are male. The age–sex bar chart shows how the deaths are distributed across the age groups, with younger men being particularly vulnerable. The deaths in the youngest age groups will most likely be accidents where the intent is undetermined, rather than suicides.

MAP 4   ALL SUICIDE/UNDETERMINED DEATHS

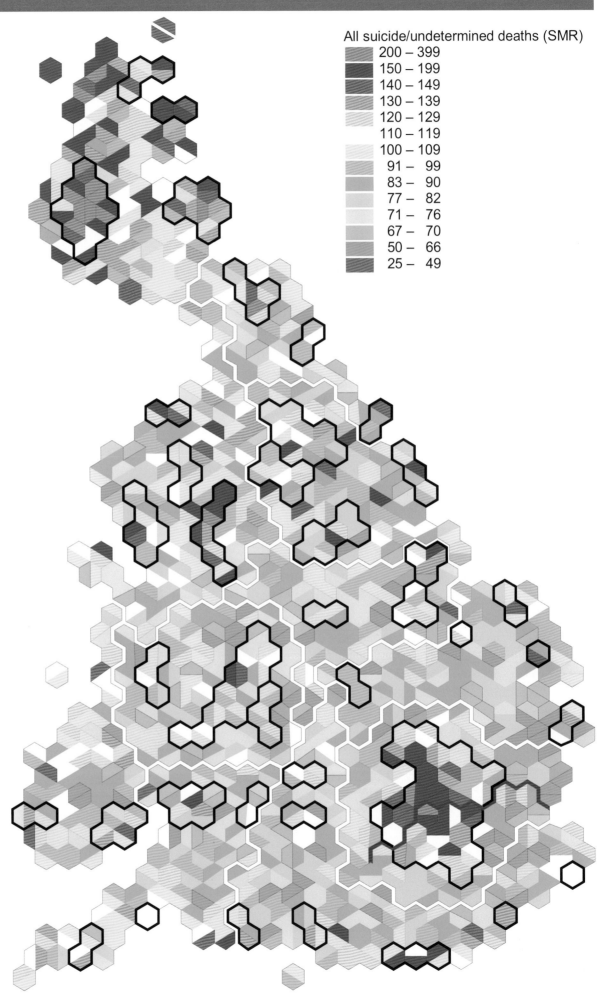

All suicide/undetermined deaths (SMR)

	200 – 399
	150 – 199
	140 – 149
	130 – 139
	120 – 129
	110 – 119
	100 – 109
	91 – 99
	83 – 90
	77 – 82
	71 – 76
	67 – 70
	50 – 66
	25 – 49

5   ALL EXTERNAL DEATHS

External causes of deaths are those due to accidents or unintentional injury, suicide or self-inflicted injury, homicide or assault injury and 'intent not able to be determined' (for example when it is not clear if a death was suicide or an accident). This category also includes deaths due to legal intervention or acts of war.

454,102 cases

3.06% of all deaths

average age = 54.0

male:female ratio = 61:39

The most striking feature of the map of all deaths attributed to causes external to the body is the higher rates found in Scotland. As we have said previously, a small part of this excess is due to the different recording system employed north of the border leading to rates being slightly inflated in Scotland in contrast to England and Wales where rates are slightly deflated. These differences in recording do not, however, account for the bulk of the national variation observed.

Suicide, homicide and accident rates in general are higher across Scotland than in almost all of England other than in Blackpool (the city with the highest proportion of divorcees in Britain), the centre of Manchester, that part of Liverpool highlighted earlier with respect to all-cause mortality and homicide, and similar neighbourhoods in Leeds, Birmingham and half a dozen such places in London. Rates of deaths from all external causes are low in the Outer London suburbs, the Home Counties (down to the south coast) and particularly noticeably low in parts of Bristol and Sheffield. The underlying causes for this pattern are largely the amalgamation of the underlying causes for the patterns of falls, self-inflicted deaths and deaths involving motor vehicles, which account for over 60% of deaths from external causes.

Group	Causes	Map	% of cases
All external deaths	Accidental deaths due to electric current	17	0.3
	Assault by cutting	18	0.6
	Assault using firearms	20	0.2
	Other assaults	21	0.9
	Motor vehicle accidents	22	14.1
	Water transport accidents	24	0.2
	Pedal cyclist hit by vehicle	25	1.1
	Railway accidents	26	0.4
	Accidental drowning	27	1.5
	Air accidents	29	0.2
	Deaths caused by machinery	30	0.4
	Other suicide/undetermined accidents	31	6.0
	Suicide/undetermined by gases	32	4.6
	Suicide/undetermined by jumping	33	1.2
	Suicide/undetermined by hanging	34	9.2
	Suicide/undetermined by firearms	35	1.0
	Accidental poisoning	36	0.8
	Suicide/undetermined by poison	38	9.0
	Suicide/undetermined by cutting	39	0.6
	Pedestrian hit by vehicle	41	6.4
	Suicide/undetermined by drowning	42	2.7
	Fire	43	3.1
	Choking on food	45	2.0
	Hunger, thirst, exposure, neglect	50	0.2
	Other external causes	52	8.5
	During surgery, medical care	69	1.9
	Hypothermia	81	1.2
	Falls	91	21.7
			100.0

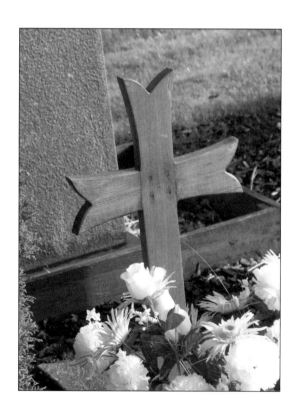

MAP 5   ALL EXTERNAL DEATHS

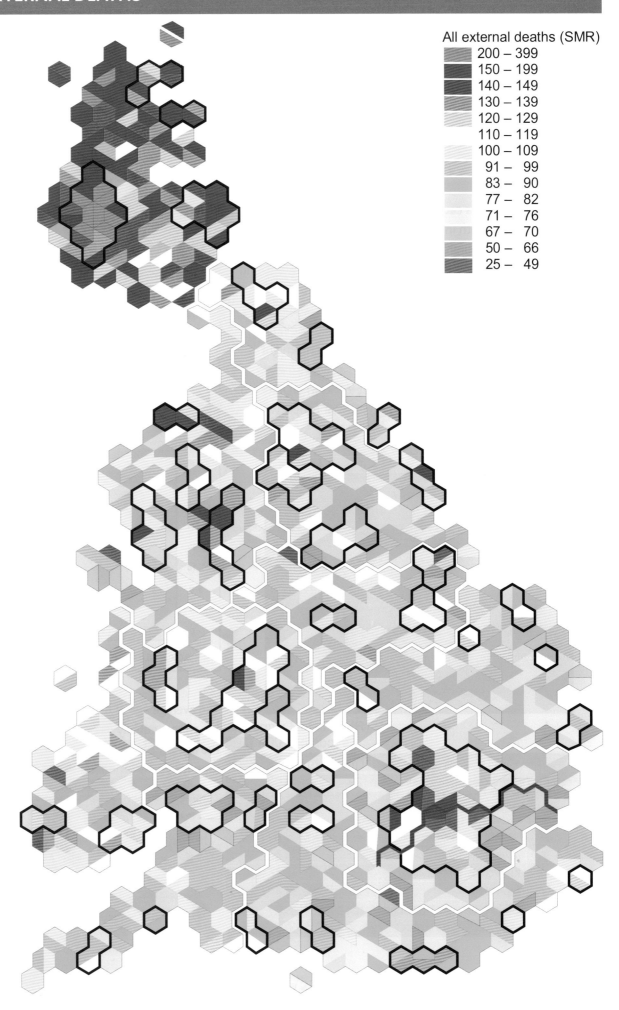

All external deaths (SMR)

	200 – 399
	150 – 199
	140 – 149
	130 – 139
	120 – 129
	110 – 119
	100 – 109
	91 – 99
	83 – 90
	77 – 82
	71 – 76
	67 – 70
	50 – 66
	25 – 49

7   ALL CANCER DEATHS

This category includes all deaths from all types of cancer, many of which are mapped individually in this atlas.

3,702,043 cases

24.96% of all deaths

average age = 70.9

male:female ratio = 52:48

This category has accounted for 3.7 million deaths over the 24 years covered in this atlas, which have been almost evenly split between males (52%) and females (48%). The average age at death is 70.9. Nearly a quarter of deaths from cancer were due to lung cancer.

Group	Causes	Map	% of cases
All cancer deaths	Cancer of brain	46	1.8
	Cervical cancer	53	1.1
	Skin cancer	54	0.9
	Leukaemia	58	2.5
	Ovarian cancer	59	2.8
	Cancer of the mouth	60	1.2
	Other neoplasms	61	5.3
	Breast cancer	62	9.0
	Lymphatic cancer	64	4.2
	Laryngeal cancer	65	0.6
	Cancer of the liver	67	1.2
	Lung cancer	68	23.6
	Cancer of gullet	71	3.9
	Pancreatic cancer	72	4.2
	Rectal cancer	74	3.8
	Other uterine cancer	76	1.0
	Unspecified neoplasms	77	11.0
	Stomach cancer	78	5.6
	Colon cancer	79	7.5
	Bladder cancer	83	3.3
	Prostate cancer	95	5.5
			100.0

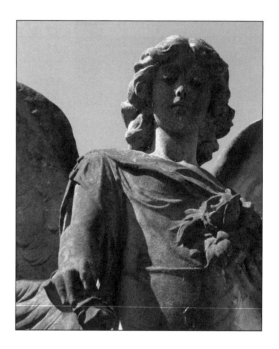

For all cancers in the south of England or in Wales, only in one part of London has a rate of 30% above the national average been recorded. In contrast, in the centres of many northern cities there are clusters of rates 30%, 40% or 50% above the national average, the most prominent being within Glasgow. Few areas in Scotland record rates below 90% of the national average. In the north of England such lower rates are only common in north Yorkshire and the more affluent parts of Lancashire. This overall pattern is largely a reflection of the smoking and poverty gradient across Britain, although there are many other causal factors implicated in cancer deaths. There is also evidence that non-smokers were more likely to migrate out of areas such as the poorer parts of Glasgow than were smokers over the course of these years, so differential migration also accounts for part of the patterns seen.

MAP 7   ALL CANCER DEATHS

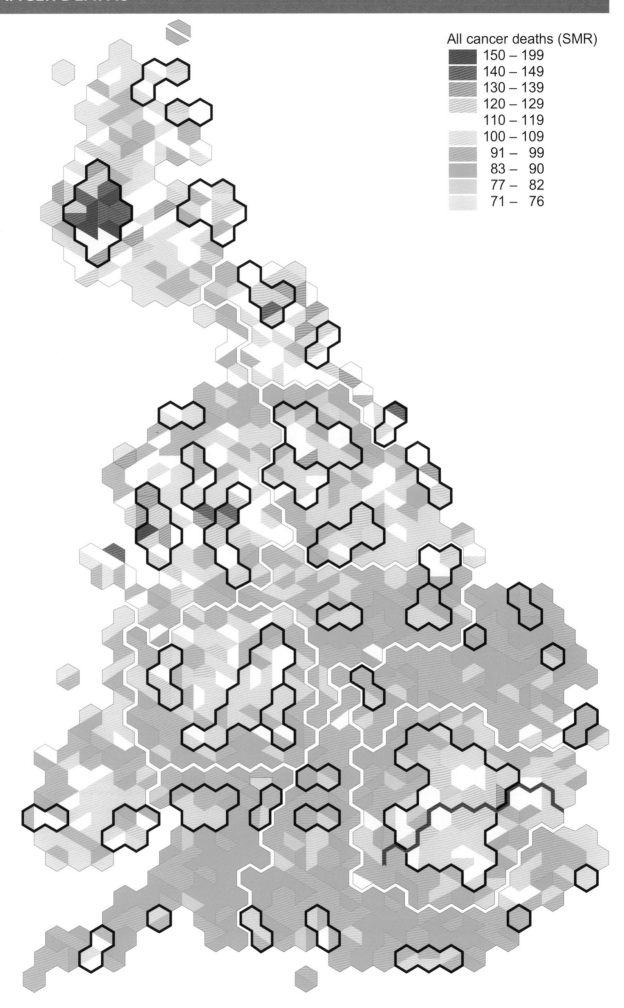

All cancer deaths (SMR)
- 150 – 199
- 140 – 149
- 130 – 139
- 120 – 129
- 110 – 119
- 100 – 109
- 91 – 99
- 83 – 90
- 77 – 82
- 71 – 76

8 ALL MENTAL DISORDER DEATHS

This category includes deaths due to drugs, alcohol and mental illnesses such as schizophrenia.

148,892 cases

1.00% of all deaths

average age = 71.7

male:female ratio = 42:58

This cause accounts for one in a hundred of all deaths. More females than males die from mental disorders (58% compared with 42%) and the average age at death is 71.7.

Which deaths should get recorded as being due to mental disorder is unclear; for example deaths due to alcohol can either be recorded as 'alcoholism' (a mental disorder) or in the category of physical morbidity (for example liver cirrhosis).

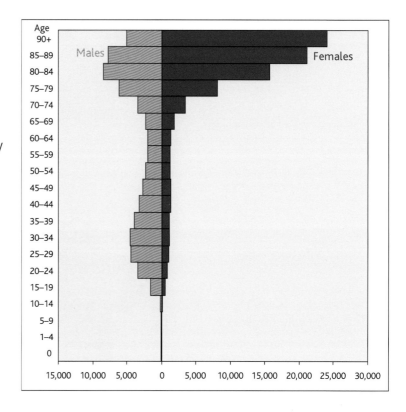

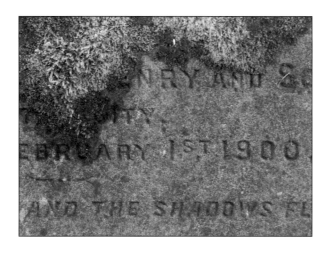

Scotland's recording of higher rates of death from these causes compared with most of England and Wales may be influenced in part by differences in the way suspected causes of death are initially recorded in that country, but as we have said before, this will only account for a small part of the differences seen north and south of that national border. By looking at the shading of neighbourhoods lying directly either side of that border it is possible to see that there is not a huge disjuncture there.

High rates of death from mental disorder follow a pattern similar to that seen for suicide, with higher rates in cities such as London, and similar causes are likely to be at play. Low rates are found in better-off cities, especially in the south.

Group	Causes	Map	% of cases
All mental disorder deaths	Deaths due to drugs	19	17.6
	Due to alcohol	40	11.4
	Other mental disorders	107	71.0
			100.0

MAP 8A (FEMALES) 8B (MALES) ALL MENTAL DISORDER DEATHS

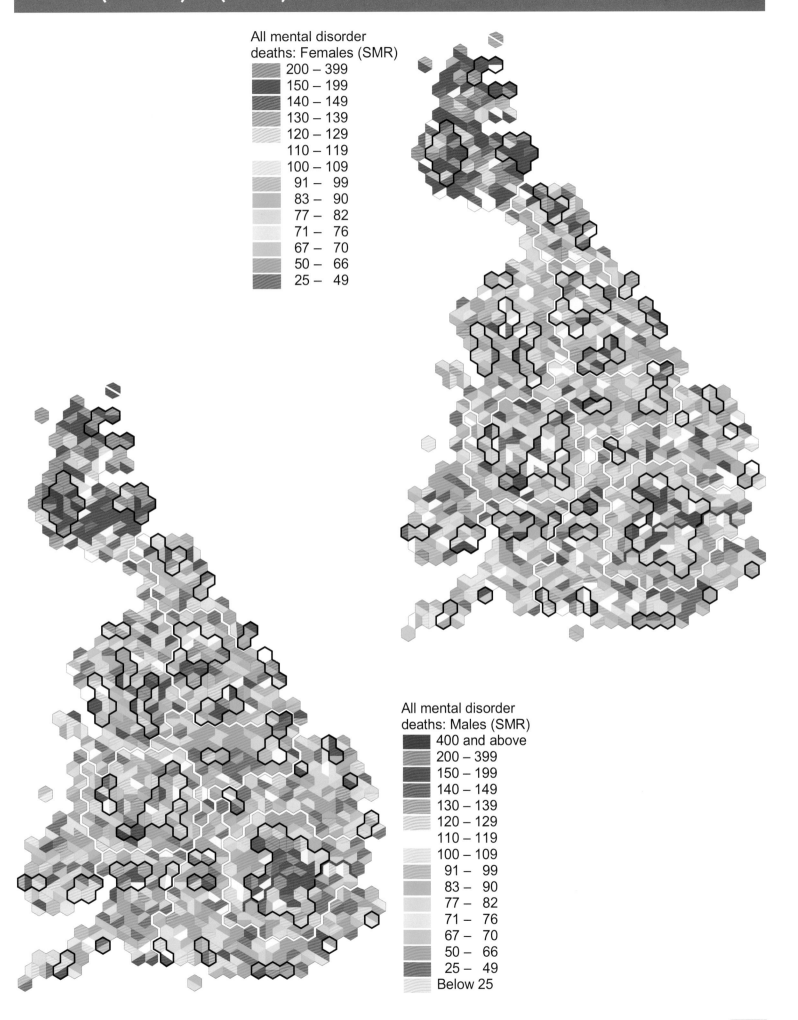

All mental disorder
deaths: Females (SMR)

- 200 – 399
- 150 – 199
- 140 – 149
- 130 – 139
- 120 – 129
- 110 – 119
- 100 – 109
- 91 – 99
- 83 – 90
- 77 – 82
- 71 – 76
- 67 – 70
- 50 – 66
- 25 – 49

All mental disorder
deaths: Males (SMR)

- 400 and above
- 200 – 399
- 150 – 199
- 140 – 149
- 130 – 139
- 120 – 129
- 110 – 119
- 100 – 109
- 91 – 99
- 83 – 90
- 77 – 82
- 71 – 76
- 67 – 70
- 50 – 66
- 25 – 49
- Below 25

9   ALL CARDIOVASCULAR DEATHS

This category includes all causes of death connected with the heart and the cardiovascular system which distributes blood throughout the body.

6,603,640 cases

44.52% of all deaths

average age = 76.7

male:female ratio = 48:52

Over 6.6 million people died from cardiovascular diseases between 1981 and 2004 inclusive – 44% of all deaths. More than half (56%) of these deaths were due to heart attacks and chronic heart disease. The deaths are fairly evenly split between males and females.

This most important group of causes of death in terms of absolute numbers of people dying before very old age is also the group with one of the clearest geographical patterns. Risks rise as you move north and into cities, with the peak being within the very centre of Glasgow. Risks are lowest in parts of Oxford and Reading; in Surrey; within London to the west by the banks of the Thames; and in the commuting lands between Bristol and Southampton.

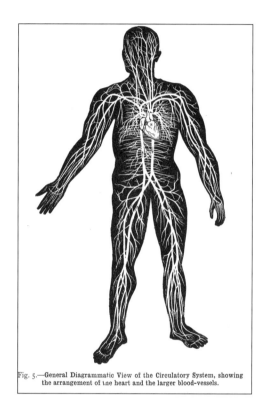

Fig. 5.—General Diagrammatic View of the Circulatory System, showing the arrangement of the heart and the larger blood-vessels.

Group	Causes	Map	% of cases
All cardiovascular deaths	Rheumatic heart disease	75	0.8
	Pulmonary circulatory disorders	82	1.5
	Heart attack and chronic heart disease	84	56.7
	Hypertensive disease	86	1.4
	Aortic anuerysm	89	3.3
	Other circulatory disorders	92	3.8
	Cerebrovascular disease	98	25.8
	Other heart disease	100	5.3
	Atherosclerosis	108	1.4
			100.0

The spatial distribution as a whole is almost smooth enough that it could be mistaken for a topographic landscape, were London a hill rather than in a hollow. It is the variations shown here that account for the largest part of the national variation in all-cause mortality, and underlying these variations are social, economic and historical patterns that have long antecedents. In terms of cardiovascular mortality, the north–south divide that runs from the Bristol Channel, skirting under Coventry, through the north of Nottingham and entering the sea with the Humber estuary just south of Hull, is clear.

MAP 9   ALL CARDIOVASCULAR DEATHS

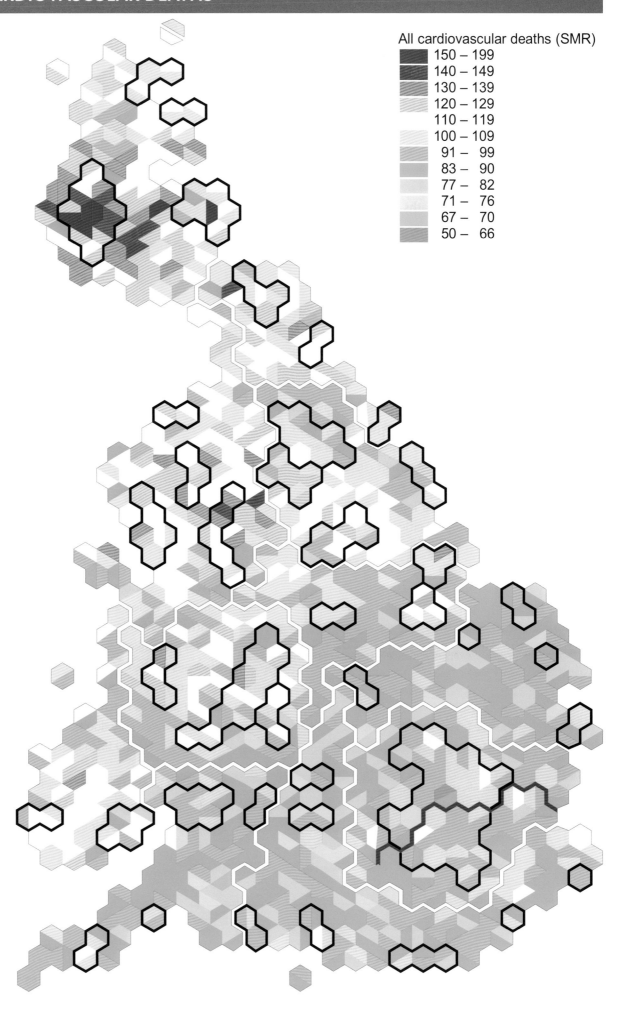

All cardiovascular deaths (SMR)

	150 – 199
	140 – 149
	130 – 139
	120 – 129
	110 – 119
	100 – 109
	91 – 99
	83 – 90
	77 – 82
	71 – 76
	67 – 70
	50 – 66

11 CONDITIONS OF THE PERINATAL PERIOD

'Perinatal' refers to conditions of the newborn, more specifically, the deaths of babies from the seventh month of pregnancy until the baby is a week old. This is a residual category of the broader category 'perinatal conditions'. For the death rates here, the conditions start in the perinatal period but the actual deaths can occur after the perinatal period (reflected in the average age of death).

29,696 cases

0.20% of all deaths

average age = 5 months

male:female ratio = 59:41

From the most privileged neighbourhoods of the Home Counties to the worst-off northern inner cities and almost all of Scotland, an infant's chances of dying from these conditions varies more than tenfold. All of the neighbourhoods with SMRs of 200 or above are in Scotland, apart from the Birmingham neighbourhood of West Bromwich Central. These deaths do not include sudden death, cause unknown, or deaths from congenital defects.

A quarter of these deaths are a result of low birthweight. A birthweight below 2,500g (5lb 8oz) is considered to be low. Low birthweight may be due to the baby being born early (prematurity) or the baby may be growth retarded (small for the period it has been in the womb). Causes and associations include illnesses in the mother, her smoking, her poverty and her malnutrition. Multiple pregnancies (twins etc) also cause lower birthweight. The lower the birthweight, the higher the need for skilled medical help for the baby to survive. Low birthweight can cause cerebral palsy where there is paralysis affecting the use of arms, legs and the muscles used in speech. Low birthweight caused 2.22% of all deaths worldwide in 2002. In Britain it is responsible for a proportion 100 times smaller.

Over half of these deaths are due to trauma around the time of birth or shortly after, such as asphyxia and other respiratory distress. Before birth, a baby receives oxygen from its mother's placenta via the blood in the umbilical cord. After birth it gets oxygen from its own lungs by breathing. Difficulties during labour can cause a delay between the first stopping and the second starting. The baby then becomes short of oxygen (birth asphyxia), which can be immediately fatal. Birth trauma refers to injuries to the baby that occur during the process of birth. These can also cause brain damage by causing bleeding inside the skull and from skull fractures. Other causes account for less than a quarter of these cases.

ICD-9 codes: 760-779

ICD-10 codes: G70.2, P00-P05, P07, P10-P11, P15, P20-P28, P29.0-P29.1, P29.8, P35-P37, P39, P50, P52, P54, P59-P61, P70, P74, P76-P78, P83, P90-P92, P94, P96, Q86.0

ICD-9	ICD-9 name	% of cases	ICD-10	ICD-10 name	% of cases
765	Disorders relating to short gestation and unspecified low birthweight	25.2	P07	Disorders related to short gestation and low birth weight, not elsewhere classified	9.0
768	Intra-uterine hypoxia and birth asphyxia	11.1			
769	Respiratory distress syndrome	20.4	P22	Respiratory distress of newborn	5.1
770	Other respiratory conditions of foetus and newborn	15.0	P27	Chronic respiratory disease originating in the perinatal period	20.0
			P36	Bacterial sepsis of newborn	8.9
772	Foetal and neonatal haemorrhage	5.9			
			P77	Necrotising enterocolitis of foetus and newborn	14.0
	Other causes in group	22.4		Other causes in group	43.0
		100.0			100.0

MAP 11   CONDITIONS OF THE PERINATAL PERIOD

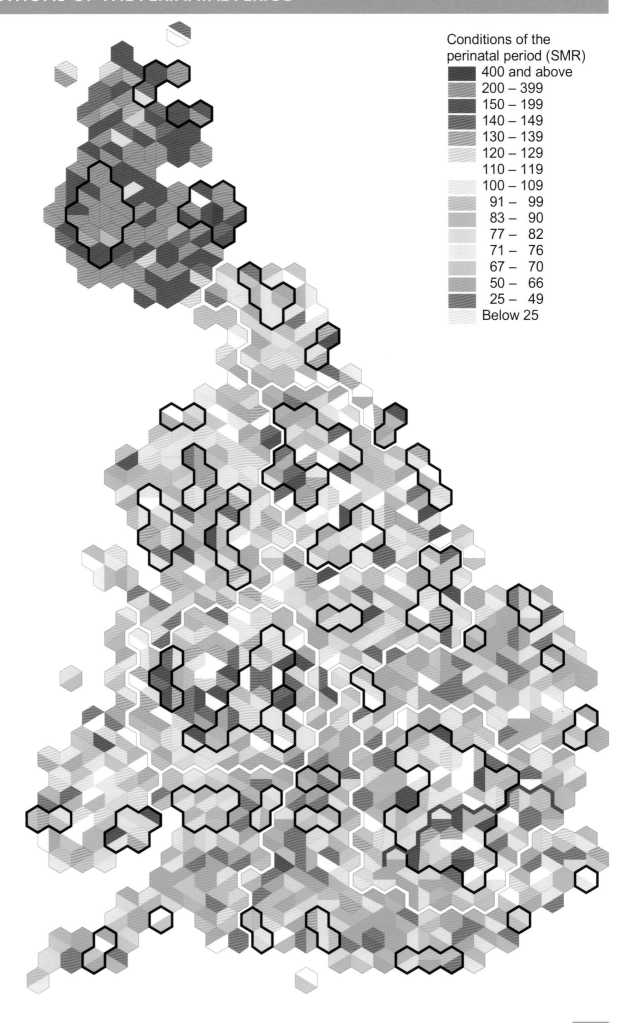

Conditions of the
perinatal period (SMR)

	400 and above
	200 – 399
	150 – 199
	140 – 149
	130 – 139
	120 – 129
	110 – 119
	100 – 109
	91 – 99
	83 – 90
	77 – 82
	71 – 76
	67 – 70
	50 – 66
	25 – 49
	Below 25

12 CONGENITAL DEFECTS OF THE NERVOUS SYSTEM

A congenital disorder is a medical condition that starts long before birth. This category includes conditions in which the brain and nervous system of a baby growing in the womb have been damaged or have not developed as they should. Most of these deaths occur in childhood, but a few occur in adulthood, resulting in an average age at which deaths occur of 13 years.

6,262 cases

0.04% of all deaths

average age = 13.0

male:female ratio = 47:53

This is a very rare cause of death, accounting for, on average, 260 deaths per year over the 24 years studied. The geographical pattern for this group of causes of death is not very strong. From the map it appears that slightly higher ratios can be seen in the northern and western parts of the country; lower rates are found within London.

These causes of death include anencephalus (the absence at birth of all or part of the brain with death occurring within days), spina bifida (a spinal cord defect) and microcephaly (a neurological disorder in which the brain is small or squashed by the skull). The word 'microcephaly' derives from the Greek for small head. Microcephaly may be congenital or it may develop in the first few years of life.

Spina bifida, which accounts for approximately a third of deaths in this category, is a condition whereby a baby is born with a damaged spinal cord due to incomplete closing of the spine around it. This can cause difficulty walking and incontinence of urine and faeces. It is a common reason for a child needing to use a wheelchair; the child is not impaired above the level of the spinal defect. Many cases of spina bifida are due to inadequate intake of folic acid by the mother; taking folic acid around the time of conception can significantly reduce the incidence of spina bifida.

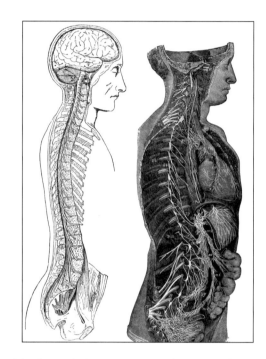

Congenital hydrocephalus, sometimes known as 'water on the brain', is when there is an abnormal accumulation of cerebrospinal fluid in the cavities of the brain, causing pressure and leading to enlargement of the head.

The remainder of deaths in this category are due to several other congenital defects of the nervous system which are often not specified further in the records.

ICD-9 codes: 740-742
ICD-10 codes: Q00-Q07

ICD-9	ICD-9 name	% of cases	ICD-10	ICD-10 name	% of cases
740	Anencephalus and similar anomalies	5.4			
741	Spina bifida	41.7	Q05	Spina bifida	31.8
742	Other congenital anomalies of nervous system	52.9	Q02	Microcephaly	13.4
			Q03	Congenital hydrocephalus	14.7
			Q04	Other congenital malformations of brain	32.6
				Other causes in group	7.5
		100.0			100.0

MAP 14   CONGENITAL HEART DEFECTS

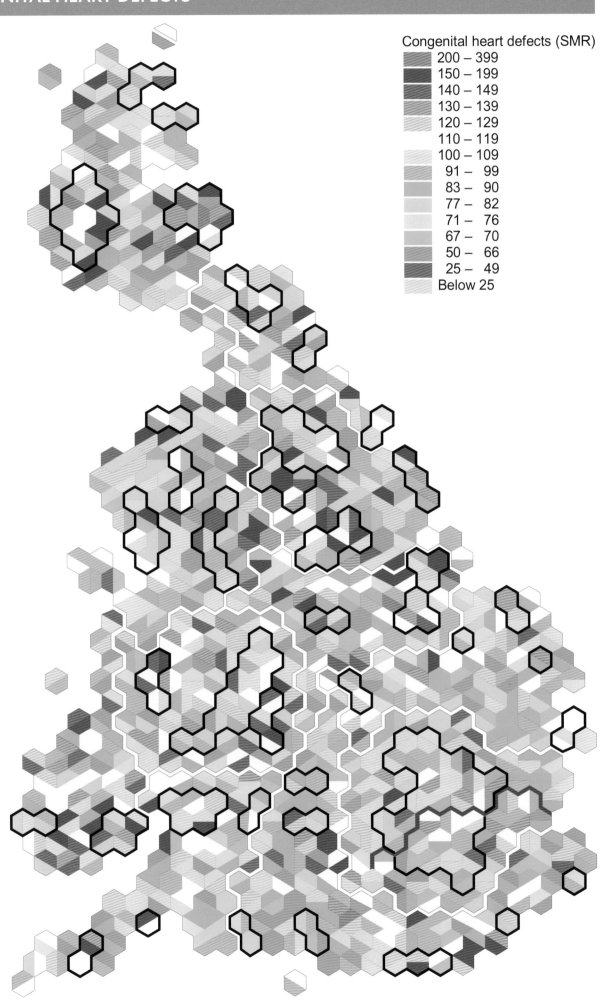

Congenital heart defects (SMR)

- 200 – 399
- 150 – 199
- 140 – 149
- 130 – 139
- 120 – 129
- 110 – 119
- 100 – 109
- 91 – 99
- 83 – 90
- 77 – 82
- 71 – 76
- 67 – 70
- 50 – 66
- 25 – 49
- Below 25

77312

15 OTHER CONGENITAL DEFECTS

A congenital disorder is a medical condition that starts at conception or in the early stages of pregnancy. This is the residual category of the broader category of congenital defects and includes all conditions other than those relating to the nervous system (Map 12) and the heart (Map 14).

19,025 cases

0.13% of all deaths

average age = 28.9

male:female ratio = 52:48

Just as with congenital heart defects (Map 14), there are wide differences between the chances of people living in different parts of the country dying due to these causes. The average age at death for this group of causes is almost 29 years but there is a very wide range around that mean. There is a north–south gradient, with Scotland and the north west tending to have higher rates, and the south of Britain lower rates.

Although these conditions start from an abnormality present long before birth, many are not diagnosed until after birth or sometimes later in life. The causes of death within this category include Down's syndrome, which in the more recent period covered by ICD-10 (used since 2000 in Scotland and 2001 in England and Wales) account for a third of all deaths in this category. Down's syndrome is a chromosomal disorder, which means that there is a change in the normal number of chromosomes (long strands of DNA containing all the genes). A baby normally has 23 pairs of chromosomes in every cell. In the most common form of Down's syndrome there are three copies of chromosome number 21, instead of the usual two copies of it.

Down's syndrome causes relatively impaired mental functioning, abnormal appearance and often congenital heart defects and other congenital disorders. Some children die before one year old from the congenital heart defects. Overall, people with Down's syndrome have a shortened lifespan.

Down's syndrome becomes much more common in babies born to mothers over age 35 years. Other than maternal age, no other risk factors are known. Many standard pre-natal non-invasive screening tests can detect Down's syndrome, although all have a non-negligible chance of producing a false positive result suggesting that a foetus has Down's syndrome when in fact it does not.

ICD-9 codes: 743-744, 748-759
ICD-10 codes: Q30-Q35, Q37-Q41, Q43-Q45, Q54, Q60-Q68, Q73-Q82, Q84, Q85.1, Q85.8-Q85.9, Q86.8, Q87, Q89-Q93, Q96-Q99

ICD-9	ICD-9 name	% of cases	ICD-10	ICD-10 name	% of cases
748	Congenital anomalies of respiratory system	11.2			
750	Other congenital anomalies of upper alimentary tract	6.0	Q38	Other congenital malformations of tongue, mouth and pharynx	5.3
751	Other congenital anomalies of digestive system	7.4			
753	Congenital anomalies of urinary system	20.6			
			Q61	Cystic kidney disease	15.0
756	Other congenital musculoskeletal anomalies	13.1			
758	Chromosomal anomalies	19.9	Q90	Down's syndrome	32.6
759	Other and unspecified congenital anomalies	18.5	Q87	Other specified congenital malformation syndromes affecting multiple systems	9.4
	Other causes in group	3.3		Other causes in group	37.7
		100.0			100.0

MAP 15 OTHER CONGENITAL DEFECTS

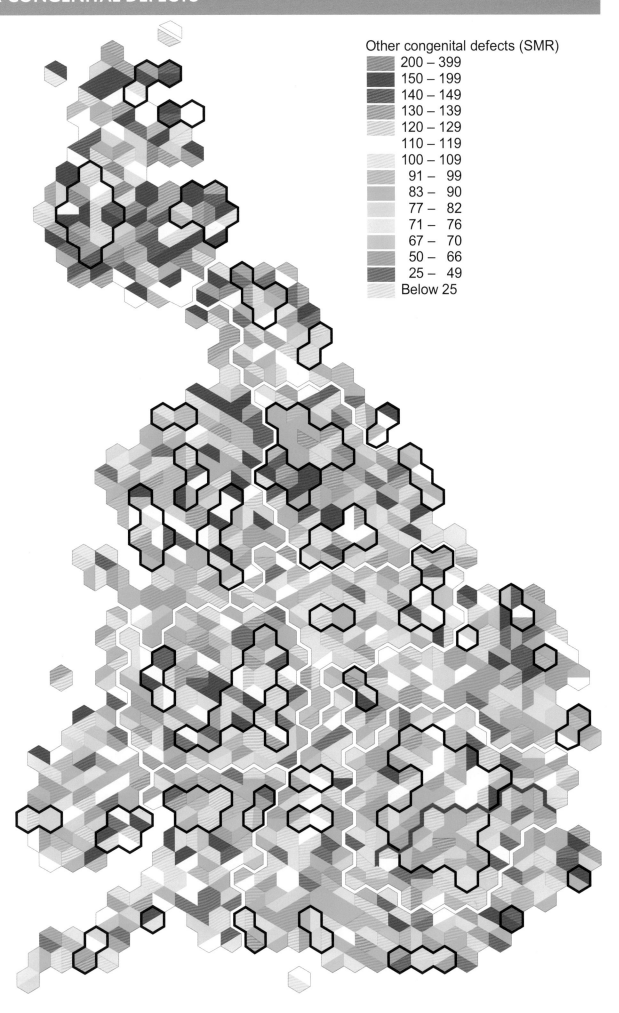

Other congenital defects (SMR)
- 200 – 399
- 150 – 199
- 140 – 149
- 130 – 139
- 120 – 129
- 110 – 119
- 100 – 109
- 91 – 99
- 83 – 90
- 77 – 82
- 71 – 76
- 67 – 70
- 50 – 66
- 25 – 49
- Below 25

16   PREGNANCY AND CHILDBIRTH

1,201 cases

0.01% of all deaths

average age = 29.8

male:female ratio = 0:100

This category can also be referred to as maternal mortality. Maternal conditions are those affecting women because they are pregnant, or when giving birth or shortly after and are due to the birth. They include haemorrhage (bleeding), infection, eclampsia, ectopic pregnancy, high blood pressure, difficulties giving birth (obstructed labour) and conditions due to abortions and miscarriages.

In much of the country rates are very low with two fifths of neighbourhoods having SMRs below 25. Twenty-one neighbourhoods have SMRs of 400 and above, with a worrying cluster of the three Birmingham neighbourhoods of Handsworth, Ladywood East and Hodge Hill West.

Maternal mortality is now a rare cause of death in the developed world. In Britain it has accounted for about 50 deaths per year over the last two decades. All maternal deaths in the UK are investigated by the Confidential Inquiry into Maternal and Child Health (CEMACH).

However, in other parts of the world this is still a prominent cause of death for women. The countries with the highest rates of death due to pregnancy and childbirth are Sierra Leone, Angola and Afghanistan (see www.worldmapper.org).

In the ICD-10 time period a quarter of deaths in this category are indirect, that is, they are pregnancy-related deaths of patients with a pre-existing or newly developed health problem.

Indirect causes are conditions such as malaria, anaemia and HIV/AIDS that complicate pregnancy or are aggravated by it.

The maternal mortality ratio (MMR) is the ratio of the number of maternal deaths per 100,000 live births. It is used as a measure of the quality of a health care system as high rates of maternal mortality reflect poor nutrition and health care. The decline in maternal deaths in rich countries over the past century has been due to improved infection control, the use of Caesarean section, fluid management and blood transfusion, and improved pre-natal care.

ICD-9 codes: 630-635, 637-644, 646-648, 653-663, 665-671, 673-675

ICD-10 codes: O00, O02, O04-O05, O10, O13-O16, O22-O24, O26, O30, O32-O34, O36, O41, O45-O46, O62, O67-O68, O71-O75, O85-O90, O98-O99

ICD-9	ICD-9 name	% of cases	ICD-10	ICD-10 name	% of cases
633	Ectopic pregnancy	9.0	O00	Ectopic pregnancy	7.0
642	Hypertension complicating pregnancy, childbirth and the puerperium	16.3	O14	Gestational [pregnancy-induced] hypertension with significant proteinuria	5.5
648	Other current conditions in the mother classifiable elsewhere but complicating pregnancy, childbirth and the puerperium	15.2	O99	Other maternal diseases classifiable elsewhere but complicating pregnancy, childbirth and the puerperium	25.5
			O75	Other complications of labour and delivery, not elsewhere classified	5.0
671	Venous complications in pregnancy and the puerperium	8.4			
673	Obstetrical pulmonary embolism	10.9	O88	Obstetric embolism	11.5
674	Other and unspecified complications of the puerperium, not elsewhere classified	7.4	O90	Complications of the puerperium, not elsewhere classified	7.5
	Other causes in group	32.8		Other causes in group	38.0
		100.0			100.0

MAP 16 PREGNANCY AND CHILDBIRTH

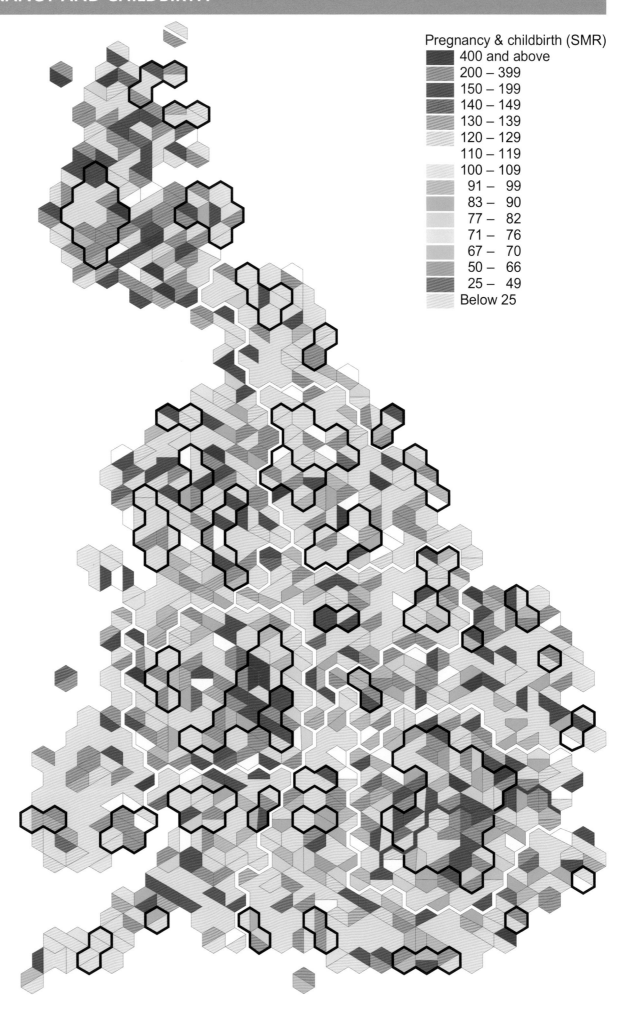

Pregnancy & childbirth (SMR)
- 400 and above
- 200 – 399
- 150 – 199
- 140 – 149
- 130 – 139
- 120 – 129
- 110 – 119
- 100 – 109
- 91 – 99
- 83 – 90
- 77 – 82
- 71 – 76
- 67 – 70
- 50 – 66
- 25 – 49
- Below 25

17 ACCIDENTAL DEATHS DUE TO ELECTRIC CURRENT

This is a sub-category of the broader category 'external' causes of death (Map 5). Approximately one person a week, usually a man, dies from this cause of death.

> 1,365 cases
>
> 0.01% of all deaths
>
> average age = 34.6
>
> male:female ratio = 87:13

Very few females die from this cause – almost nine out of ten deaths are of males. There is no apparent geographical pattern to deaths from this cause, but perhaps a slight preponderance of higher rates in the south east, possibly reflecting more construction work there.

This category covers accidental deaths from electrocutions from domestic appliances such as light fittings, water heaters, washing machines and extension cords. The reasons for the equipment causing death include faulty equipment and damaged or exposed wiring; sometimes the accident will result from someone having tampered with equipment contrary to safety advice. Power tools, such as electric drills, and gardening equipment, such as lawnmowers and hedge-trimmers, are also common causes of accidents involving an electric cable in a domestic environment.

Many deaths in this category will be deaths in the workplace; those working on farms and in the power supply industry are at particular risk. Building sites also constitute a high-risk environment in this regard. Accidents can include cranes and ladders coming into contact with power lines, and pipes, poles and vehicles that have become energised. The people working in these jobs tend to be younger males, as reflected in the statistics above.

Many of these deaths could be avoided by the implementation of appropriate safety measures and procedures.

This category does not include deaths due to lightning. Those are included in 'other external causes' of death (Map 52).

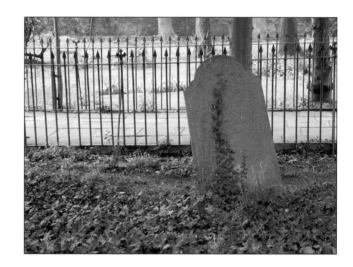

ICD-9 codes: E925
ICD-10 codes: W85-W87

ICD-9	ICD-9 name	% of cases	ICD-10	ICD-10 name	% of cases
E925	Accident caused by electric current	100.0	W85	Exposure to electric transmission lines	6.8
			W86	Exposure to other specified electric current	72.0
			W87	Exposure to unspecified electric current	21.2
		100.0			100.0

MAP 17   ACCIDENTAL DEATHS DUE TO ELECTRIC CURRENT

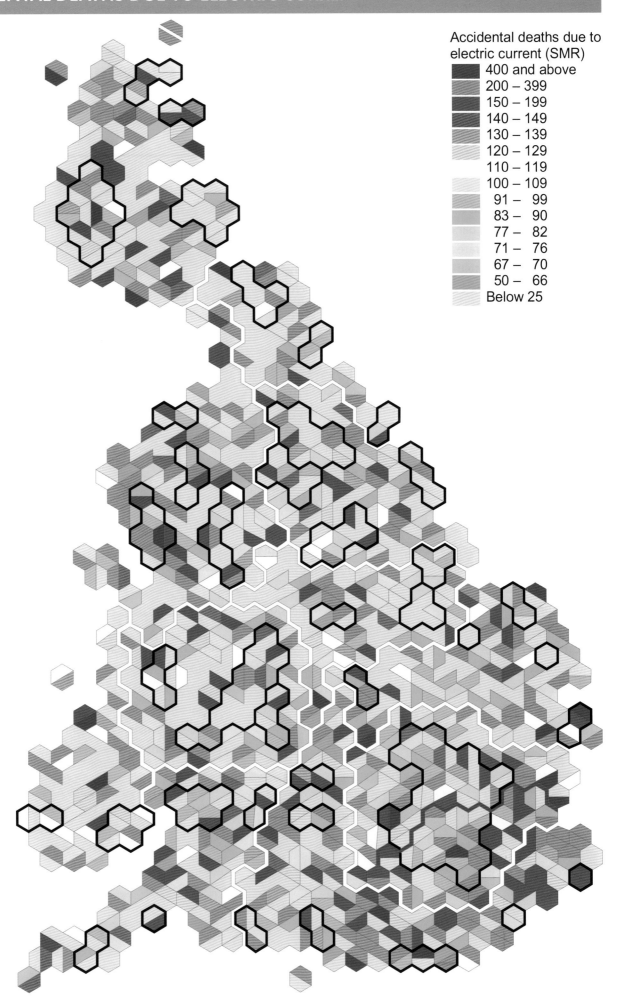

Accidental deaths due to
electric current (SMR)

- 400 and above
- 200 – 399
- 150 – 199
- 140 – 149
- 130 – 139
- 120 – 129
- 110 – 119
- 100 – 109
- 91 – 99
- 83 – 90
- 77 – 82
- 71 – 76
- 67 – 70
- 50 – 66
- Below 25

19 DEATHS DUE TO DRUGS

This category includes accidental deaths due to the use of mind-altering (psychoactive) substances for non-medical purposes, also referred to as substance misuse, drug misuse, illegal drug use and recreational drug use. Deaths due to alcohol are covered in Map 40, while deaths due to suicide/undetermined by poison are included in Map 38.

26,162 cases

0.18% of all deaths

average age = 35.0

male:female ratio = 74:26

Accidental deaths due to drugs account for three deaths a day in Britain. There is clearly a rural–urban divide with the highest rates seen in Glasgow, Brighton and London, followed by other towns and cities as well as some coastal resorts of former glory. The latter are often places in which local authorities have re-housed those whom they are obliged to accommodate under homeless persons legislation. In contrast, some remote rural areas, particularly in Scotland, have extremely low rates.

A wide range of often illegal drugs is included here (although the two most commonly used recreational drugs – alcohol and tobacco – are not included here). They include opiates (such as heroin and morphine), amphetamines, cocaine, barbiturates (sleeping pills), drugs that cause hallucinations (such as lysergic acid, LSD) and hydrocarbons ('glue sniffing'). There is often more than one drug used and alcohol is frequently also involved. This can make it difficult to attribute the cause of death to one particular drug.

Estimating mortality directly attributable to illicit drug use such as overdose death is often difficult because the drugs are illegal, stigmatised and hidden.

Deaths from diseases spread by non-sterile needles and syringes, such as Hepatitis B and C (see Map 44) and HIV/AIDS (see Map 28), are counted separately.

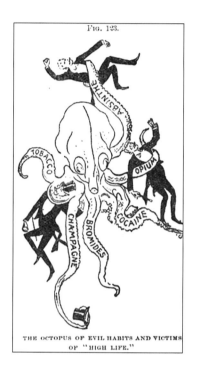

FIG. 123.

THE OCTOPUS OF EVIL HABITS AND VICTIMS OF "HIGH LIFE."

ICD-9 codes: 304, 305.1-305.9, E850-E858
ICD-10 codes: F11.0-F11.2, F12.1-F12.2, F13.1-F13.2, F14, F15.1-F15.2, F16.1-F16.2, F17.2, F18, F19.0-F19.2, X40-X44, X46

ICD-9	ICD-9 name	% of cases	ICD-10	ICD-10 name	% of cases
304	Opioid type dependence	13.8	F11.2	Dependence syndrome - opioids	24.8
305.5	Opioid abuse	7.8	F11.1	Harmful use - opioids	13.4
304.6	Other specified drug dependence	5.1	F19.2	Dependence syndrome - multiple drug use and use of other psychoactive substances	10.1
			F19.1	Harmful use - multiple drug use and use of other psychoactive substances	5.6
E850	Accidental poisoning by analgesics, antipyretics, antirheumatics	28.0	X41	Accidental poisoning by and exposure to antiepileptic, sedative-hypnotic, anti-Parkinsonism and psychotropic drugs, not elsewhere classified	6.6
E854	Accidental poisoning by other psychotropic agents	5.8	X42	Accidental poisoning by and exposure to narcotics and psychodysleptics [hallucinogens], not elsewhere classified	19.3
E858	Accidental poisoning by other drugs	14.4	X44	Accidental poisoning by and exposure to other and unspecified drugs, medicaments and biological substances	12.0
	Other causes in group	25.1		Other causes in group	8.2
		100.0			100.0

MAP 19   DEATHS DUE TO DRUGS

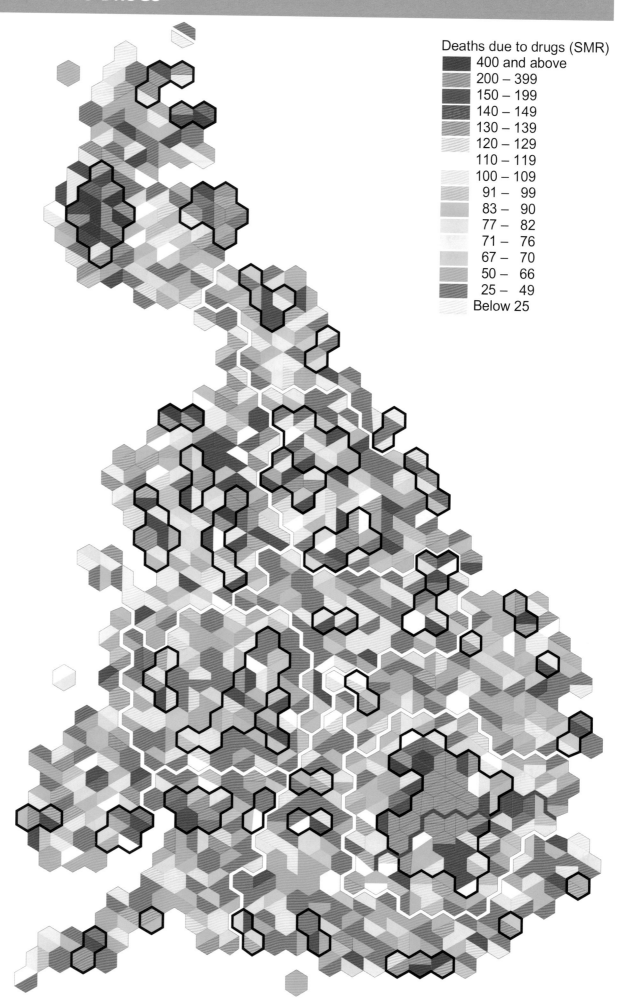

Deaths due to drugs (SMR)

- 400 and above
- 200 – 399
- 150 – 199
- 140 – 149
- 130 – 139
- 120 – 129
- 110 – 119
- 100 – 109
- 91 – 99
- 83 – 90
- 77 – 82
- 71 – 76
- 67 – 70
- 50 – 66
- 25 – 49
- Below 25

22 MOTOR VEHICLE ACCIDENTS

This category includes the majority of deaths resulting from traffic accidents. They are traffic accidents where the person who has died was a driver or passenger in a vehicle (for example, car, lorry, bus, motorcycle), and not a pedestrian or pedal cyclist.

See also Map 25 Pedal cyclist hit by vehicle and Map 41 Pedestrian hit by vehicle.

64,202 cases

0.43% of all deaths

average age = 36.9

male:female ratio = 76:24

Deaths from this cause are among the most common way that people in Britain between the ages of 15 and 34 have recently died. Below those ages they more often die while trying to cross the road as a pedestrian, or being hit by a car while cycling.

The lowest rates are generally found in the more urban areas, with London, Newcastle, Greater Manchester and Cardiff having particularly low rates.

In comparison, higher rates are more often found in rural areas, where car use is more necessary, pavements and lighting are often poorer or missing, and average speeds are higher. The highest death rates from this cause are found in the north of Scotland.

Three quarters of the victims of this cause of death are males, most of them in their teens, twenties and thirties. However, people of all ages, young and old, die from this cause.

ICD-9 codes: E810, E811.0, E812.0-E812.4, E812.8-E812.9, E813.0-E813.3, E813.5, E813.8-E813.9, E814.0-E814.3, E814.5, E814.8-E814.9, E815.0-E815.3, E815.5, E815.8-E815.9, E816.0-E816.3, E816.8-E816.9, E817.0-E817.2, E817.4, E817.8-E817.9, E818.0-E818.4, E818.8-E818.9, E819.0-E819.3, E819.8-E819.9, E821.0-E821.3, E821.8-E821.9, E822.0-E822.3, E822.8-E822.9, E823.0-E823.3, E823.8, E824.0-E824.1, E824.8-E824.9, E825.0-E825.3, E825.8-E825.9

ICD-10 codes: V20-V29, V33-V34, V37-V40, V42-V49, V53-V54, V57-V60, V63-V64, V67-V69, V73-V74, V77-V79, V80.4-V80.5, V84-V89

ICD-9	ICD-9 name	% of cases	ICD-10	ICD-10 name	% of cases
E812.0	Other motor vehicle traffic accident involving collision with another motor vehicle - Driver of motor vehicle other than motorcycle	25.0	V43.5	Car occupant injured in collision with car, pick-up truck or van - Driver injured in traffic accident	10.0
E812.1	Other motor vehicle traffic accident involving collision with another motor vehicle - Passenger in motor vehicle other than motorcycle	12.9	V44.5	Car occupant injured in collision with heavy transport vehicle or bus - Driver injured in traffic accident	5.7
E812.2	Other motor vehicle traffic accident involving collision with another motor vehicle - Motorcyclist	12.8	V23.4	Motorcycle rider injured in collision with car, pick-up truck or van - Driver injured in traffic accident	9.4
E815.0	Other motor vehicle traffic accident involving collision on the highway - Driver of motor vehicle other than motorcycle	7.1	V49.4	Car occupant injured in other and unspecified transport accidents - Driver injured in collision with other and unspecified motor vehicles in traffic accident	7.3
E816.0	Motor vehicle traffic accident due to loss of control, without collision on the highway - Driver of motor vehicle other than motorcycle	5.4	V49.9	Car occupant injured in other and unspecified transport accidents - Car occupant [any] injured in unspecified traffic accident	9.8
E819.9	Motor vehicle traffic accident of unspecified nature - Unspecified person	10.7	V47.5	Car occupant injured in collision with fixed or stationary object - Driver injured in traffic accident	12.6
	Other causes in group	26.1		Other causes in group	45.2
		100.0			100.0

MAP 22A (FEMALES) 22B (MALES)   MOTOR VEHICLE ACCIDENTS

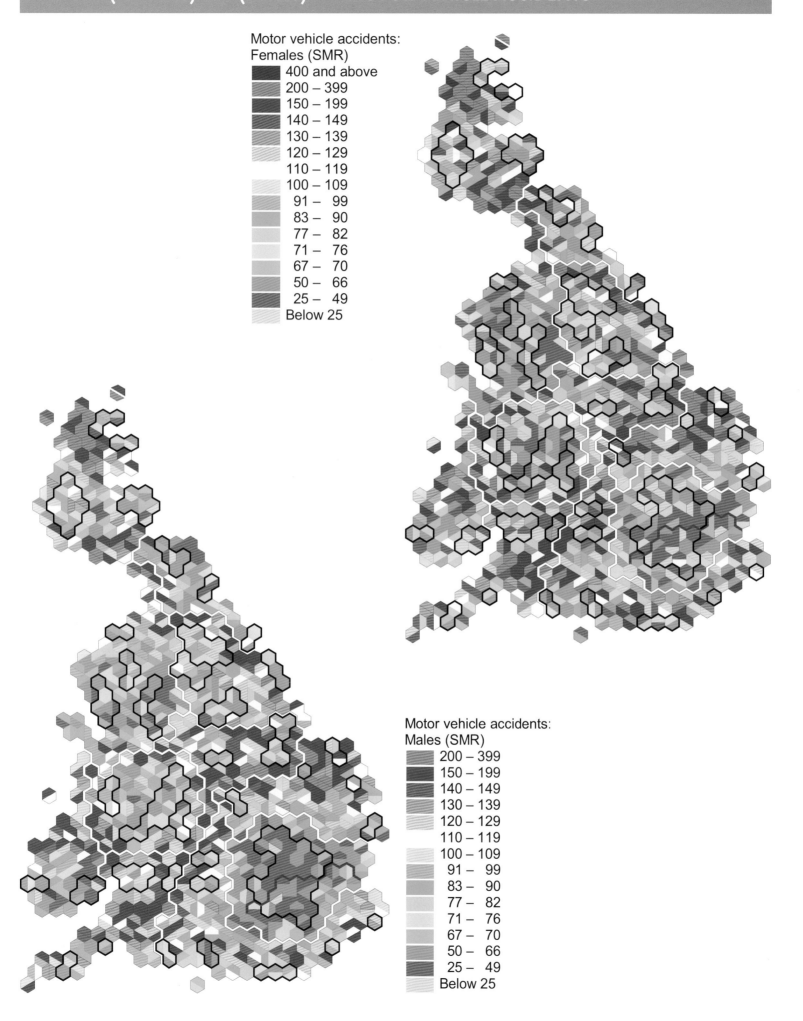

Motor vehicle accidents:
Females (SMR)
- 400 and above
- 200 – 399
- 150 – 199
- 140 – 149
- 130 – 139
- 120 – 129
- 110 – 119
- 100 – 109
- 91 – 99
- 83 – 90
- 77 – 82
- 71 – 76
- 67 – 70
- 50 – 66
- 25 – 49
- Below 25

Motor vehicle accidents:
Males (SMR)
- 200 – 399
- 150 – 199
- 140 – 149
- 130 – 139
- 120 – 129
- 110 – 119
- 100 – 109
- 91 – 99
- 83 – 90
- 77 – 82
- 71 – 76
- 67 – 70
- 50 – 66
- 25 – 49
- Below 25

23   MENINGITIS

9,982 cases

0.07% of all deaths

average age = 37.2

male:female ratio = 51:49

Meningitis is inflammation of the meninges, the lining surrounding the brain and spinal cord. It can be caused by bacteria, viruses, fungi and amoeba. One of the most common forms is meningococcal meningitis. Meningococcal infections can also cause septicaemia (blood poisoning). Viral meningitis is less severe than bacterial meningitis, which is always associated with serious and severe illness.

The general geographical pattern here is for urban areas to have higher rates. These urban areas are surrounded by neighbourhoods with rates near the national average, which in turn lie next to more suburban and rural areas with low rates. Sometimes the poorer parts of cities can be seen more often to have higher rates, such as in the east of London.

The lowest rates tend to be found in the more remote and/or rural parts of Britain. Meningitis is an infectious disease and can cluster where people live in close proximity, for example among students living in halls of residence. There are, however, some obvious anomalies to this general pattern. Much of Birmingham has rates around the national average, with rates as low as half the average in the Sutton area. Similarly, the eastern half of Dundee, parts of Leeds, and much of Norwich have lower than average rates. Thirty per cent of deaths from meningitis were of children and infants below the age of five.

Meningitis can kill, sometimes within hours, or cause permanent brain damage. The brain damage can often affect subsequent mental ability severely; it may also cause spasticity or paralysis of one or more limbs. Other long-term effects can include recurrent epileptic fits and deafness. Several bacteria can cause meningitis, and vaccines are available for some of them. Mortality can be high without the quick use of appropriate antibiotics.

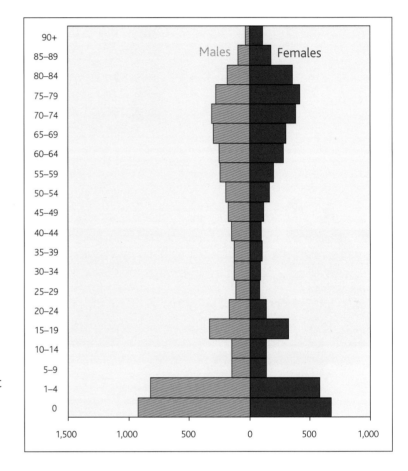

This disease affects males and females equally. Everyone is potentially at risk from meningitis but the very young are most vulnerable. Meningitis tends to be more common where there is overcrowding, poverty and malnutrition.

ICD-9 codes: 036, 320, 322
ICD-10 codes: A39, G00, G03

ICD-9	ICD-9 name	% of cases	ICD-10	ICD-10 name	% of cases
036	Meningococcal infection	38.8	A39	Meningococcal infection	39.3
320	Bacterial meningitis	38.4	G00	Bacterial meningitis, not elsewhere classified	36.2
322	Meningitis of unspecified cause	22.8	G03	Meningitis due to other and unspecified causes	24.5
		100.0			100.0

MAP 23   MENINGITIS

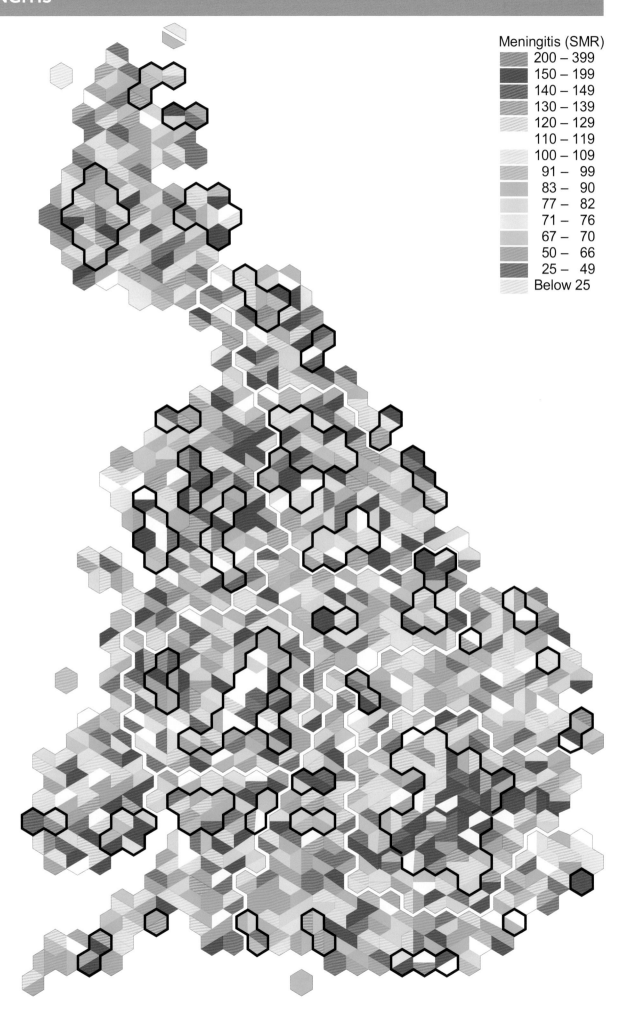

Meningitis (SMR)
200 – 399
150 – 199
140 – 149
130 – 139
120 – 129
110 – 119
100 – 109
91 – 99
83 – 90
77 – 82
71 – 76
67 – 70
50 – 66
25 – 49
Below 25

24 WATER TRANSPORT ACCIDENTS

These deaths include accidents involving some form of water transport.

Deaths due to accidental drowning that do not involve water transport are covered in Map 27 Accidental drowning. See also Map 42 Suicide/undetermined by drowning.

1,047 cases

0.01% of all deaths

average age = 38.1

male:female ratio = 92:8

This is a relatively rare cause of death – on average there has been less than one death per week. However, we can still see the geographical pattern that we would expect for this cause with deaths clustered around coastal areas. It should be noted that the deaths mapped here are coded according to the residence of the deceased, not their place of death. Those who live near the coast are more likely to work in and to participate in water-based leisure activities and are thus at more risk of dying from this cause as a result. More than nine out of ten of these deaths are of males.

It is estimated that some 450,000 boats are kept in the UK (British Marine Federation); the majority of these will be for leisure purposes. The type of vessels used include yachts, small sailboats, motor boats, power boats, jetskis, rowing boats and canoes. As well in coastal waters, boats are also used on lakes, rivers and canals. There is no legal requirement for a civilian leisure vessel under 20m in length to be registered or for the person in charge of it to be qualified or competent.

Alcohol is involved in many accidents of this nature. Most harbours have byelaws banning people from taking out a boat while under the influence of alcohol. There is legislation regarding alcohol and drug limits as well as a testing regime for professional seamen (since March 2004) in line with those that apply on the roads; at time of writing the Department for Transport had just published the responses to a consultation paper on extending the legislation to non-professional mariners.

Occupational groups that may be at risk of this cause of death include fishermen and dock workers as well as those working on container ships, oil tankers, ferries, water buses and cruise ships. A study by Roberts (2002) showed that merchant seafaring and trawler fishing are the most hazardous of all occupations and that many of the deaths of people in these occupations are caused by work-related accidents.

Roberts, S.E. (2002) 'Hazardous occupations in Great Britain', *Lancet*, vol 360, pp 543–4.

ICD-9 codes: E830-E838
ICD-10 codes: V90-V94

ICD-9	ICD-9 name	% of cases	ICD-10	ICD-10 name	% of cases
E830	Accident to watercraft causing submersion	44.6	V90	Accident to watercraft causing drowning and submersion	21.6
E831	Accident to watercraft causing other injury	6.3			
E832	Other accidental submersion or drowning in water transport accident	28.6	V92	Water-transport-related drowning and submersion without accident to watercraft	43.1
			V93	Accident on board watercraft without accident to watercraft, not causing drowning and submersion	20.6
E838	Other and unspecified water transport accident	12.3	V94	Other and unspecified water transport accidents	9.8
	Other causes in group	8.2		Other causes in group	4.9
		100.0			100.0

MAP 24   WATER TRANSPORT ACCIDENTS

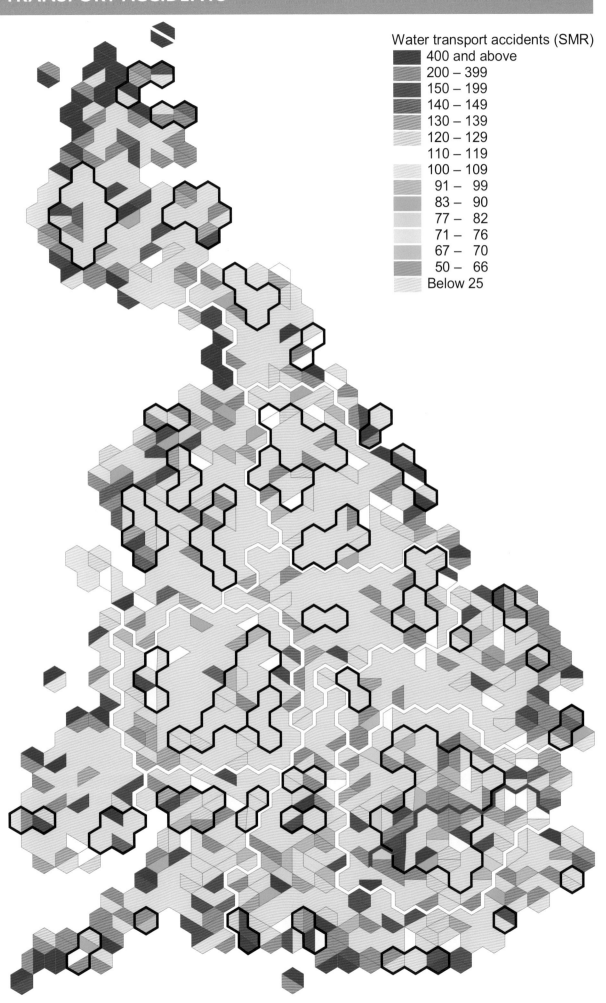

Water transport accidents (SMR)

- 400 and above
- 200 – 399
- 150 – 199
- 140 – 149
- 130 – 139
- 120 – 129
- 110 – 119
- 100 – 109
- 91 – 99
- 83 – 90
- 77 – 82
- 71 – 76
- 67 – 70
- 50 – 66
- Below 25

25   PEDAL CYCLIST HIT BY VEHICLE

This category comes under the broader category of 'external' causes of death and includes deaths to cyclists.

See also Map 22 Motor vehicle accidents and Map 41 Pedestrian hit by vehicle.

4,822 cases

0.03% of all deaths

average age = 38.4

male:female ratio = 83:17

This cause of death is far more common for males than females. The geography for this cause of death shows that rates are higher in rural areas, which may be accounted for by narrow, unlit rural roads and a lack of cycle lanes.

These deaths can result from a variety of types of collision – with other road users such as cars, lorries or buses. Cyclists also collide with other cyclists, pedestrians or stationary objects (such as lamp posts or other street furniture). Accidents do not always happen on the road itself. Particularly for young children, collisions can occur when cars are reversing on private driveways and the child on the bicycle has not been seen in the rear view mirror (or the driver has not used their mirror). Many accidents also occur 'off road', on cycle tracks or mountain bike trails. Some accidents are classed as 'noncollision', more commonly referred to as 'falling off'.

According to the Department for Transport, 10% of all accidents involving cyclists occur at roundabouts; pedal cycle fatal accident rates at roundabouts are 14 times those of cars. Often car drivers do not see bicycles as they focus on more frequent and (for them) major dangers. The design of roundabouts can improve the safety of cyclists as well as drivers. The first roundabout was constructed in Letchworth in 1910.

Bicycle helmets and cycle lanes are other strategies for improving safety for cyclists, although the effectiveness of both is debated.

ICD-9 codes: E812.6, E813.6, E814.6, E815.6, E818.6, E819.6, E821.6, E822.6, E826.1
ICD-10 codes: V10-V14, V16-V19

ICD-9	ICD-9 name	% of cases	ICD-10	ICD-10 name	% of cases
E813.6	Motor vehicle traffic accident involving collision with other vehicle – Pedal cyclist	85.2	V13.4	Pedal cyclist injured in collision with car, pick-up truck or van – Driver injured in traffic accident	36.6
			V14.4	Pedal cyclist injured in collision with heavy transport vehicle or bus – Driver injured in traffic accident	18.4
			V19.4	Pedal cyclist injured in other and unspecified transport accidents – Driver injured in collision with other and unspecified motor vehicles in traffic accident	11.2
E826.1	Pedal cycle accident – Pedal cyclist	13.6	V18	Pedal cyclist injured in noncollision transport accident	16.6
			V19.9	Pedal cyclist injured in other and unspecified transport accidents – Pedal cyclist [any] injured in unspecified traffic accident	8.2
	Other causes in group	1.2		Other causes in group	9.0
		100.0			100.0

MAP 25 PEDAL CYCLIST HIT BY VEHICLE

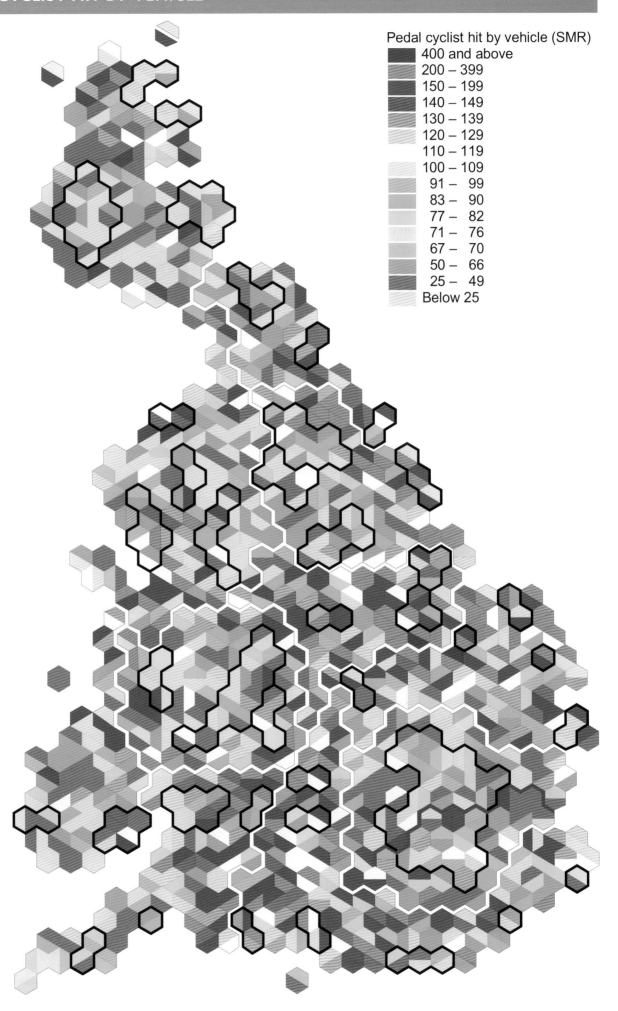

Pedal cyclist hit by vehicle (SMR)
- 400 and above
- 200 – 399
- 150 – 199
- 140 – 149
- 130 – 139
- 120 – 129
- 110 – 119
- 100 – 109
- 91 – 99
- 83 – 90
- 77 – 82
- 71 – 76
- 67 – 70
- 50 – 66
- 25 – 49
- Below 25

27 ACCIDENTAL DROWNING

This category includes accidental deaths due to drowning, whether that is in a bath, a garden pond, a lake or the sea.

See also Map 42 Suicide/undetermined by drowning and Map 24 Water transport accidents.

6,804 cases

0.05% of all deaths

average age = 38.6

male:female ratio = 76:24

For males, rates are somewhat higher in the south west of England and south Wales, where coastal waters tend to be warmer thereby encouraging more people to swim.

Three quarters of deaths due to accidental drowning are of males. Men aged 15–44 account for over one third of all deaths by accidental drowning.

Very young children and older people are those most likely to drown in the bath. Many other people who die due to accidental drowning do so because they cannot swim. However, many swimmers drown, particularly in natural water features such as lakes and rivers, because they overestimate their swimming ability.

When a person is submerged in water their lungs fill up with water and so the amount of oxygen in the bloodstream rapidly falls and the person loses consciousness. It can sometimes be difficult to establish whether drowning was accidental or whether foul play or suicide was involved. A person, and particularly young children, can drown in a few centimetres of water.

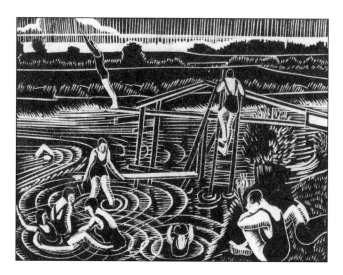

Drowning victims include the poet Percy Shelley, and Mary Jo Kopechne, who died in a car accident involving US Senator Ted Kennedy at Chappaquiddick in 1969.

ICD-9 codes: E910
ICD-10 codes: W65-W70, W73-W74

ICD-9	ICD-9 name	% of cases	ICD-10	ICD-10 name	% of cases
E910	Accidental drowning and submersion	100.0	W65	Drowning and submersion while in bath-tub	18.0
			W69	Drowning and submersion while in natural water	30.4
			W70	Drowning and submersion following fall into natural water	18.1
			W73	Other specified drowning and submersion	10.1
			W74	Unspecified drowning and submersion	17.1
				Other causes in group	6.3
		100.0			100.0

MAP 27A (FEMALES) 27B (MALES)   ACCIDENTAL DROWNING

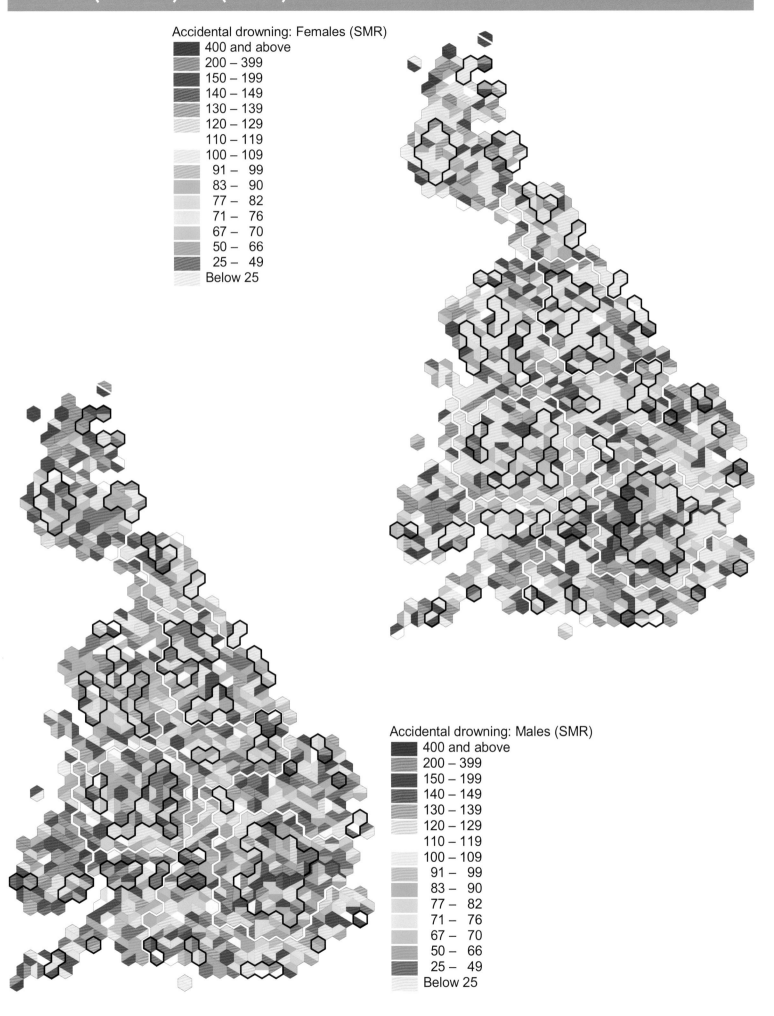

Accidental drowning: Females (SMR)

- 400 and above
- 200 – 399
- 150 – 199
- 140 – 149
- 130 – 139
- 120 – 129
- 110 – 119
- 100 – 109
- 91 – 99
- 83 – 90
- 77 – 82
- 71 – 76
- 67 – 70
- 50 – 66
- 25 – 49
- Below 25

Accidental drowning: Males (SMR)

- 400 and above
- 200 – 399
- 150 – 199
- 140 – 149
- 130 – 139
- 120 – 129
- 110 – 119
- 100 – 109
- 91 – 99
- 83 – 90
- 77 – 82
- 71 – 76
- 67 – 70
- 50 – 66
- 25 – 49
- Below 25

28 HIV DISEASE INFECTIONS

This category covers HIV (human immunodeficiency virus), the virus that causes AIDS (Acquired Immunodeficiency Syndrome), plus other deaths caused by other immunodeficiencies. Under ICD-9 about half of all deaths in this category were due to HIV. Under ICD-10 (since 2000/01) four fifths of deaths in this category were due to HIV. The increase is due to rising cases of HIV over time.

> 7,061 cases
>
> 0.05% of all deaths
>
> average age = 39.3
>
> male:female ratio = 81:19

Male and female deaths are mapped separately as the rates are so different (see also the age–sex bar chart). The highest SMRs are found in Inner London, Edinburgh (at one time labelled the 'drugs capital of Europe') and Dundee.

Over 800 of these deaths were due to haemophiliacs (who are male) contracting HIV through contaminated blood products (www.taintedblood.info). The development of antiretroviral drugs delays the onset of AIDS, thus prolonging life.

HIV/AIDS was first identified in the USA in 1981, coincidentally the first year of data included in this atlas. The total number of deaths thus includes all deaths that have ever occurred from this cause in Britain.

AIDS is caused by the human immunodeficiency virus (HIV), which slowly destroys the body's defences against diseases (the immune system). When this has happened, you have AIDS, and certain infections and cancers can easily develop and be fatal. HIV is spread sexually, in semen and other genital secretions, and the person's blood is also infectious. Mothers can infect their babies both during vaginal delivery and by breast-feeding.

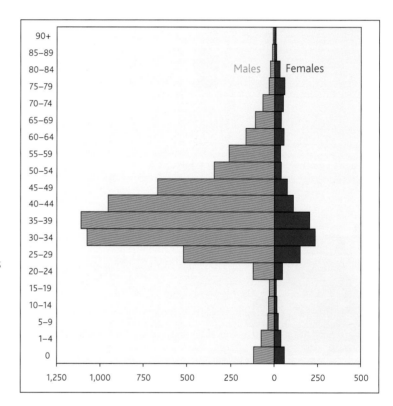

People are infectious any time after the initial infection with HIV, long before AIDS occurs.

ICD-9 codes: 042-044, 279
ICD-10 codes: B20-B24, D80-D84, D89.8-D89.9

ICD-9	ICD-9 name	% of cases	ICD-10	ICD-10 name	% of cases
042	Human immunodeficiency virus [HIV] disease	43.9	B20	Human immunodeficiency virus [HIV] disease resulting in infectious and parasitic diseases	47.1
			B21	Human immunodeficiency virus [HIV] disease resulting in malignant neoplasms	8.9
			B22	Human immunodeficiency virus [HIV] disease resulting in other specified diseases	6.5
			B23	Human immunodeficiency virus [HIV] disease resulting in other conditions	10.5
			B24	Unspecified human immunodeficiency virus [HIV] disease	9.0
279	Disorders involving the immune mechanism	49.9	D84	Other immunodeficiencies	8.9
	Other causes in group	6.2		Other causes in group	9.1
		100.0			100.0

MAP 28A (FEMALES) 28B (MALES)   HIV DISEASE INFECTIONS

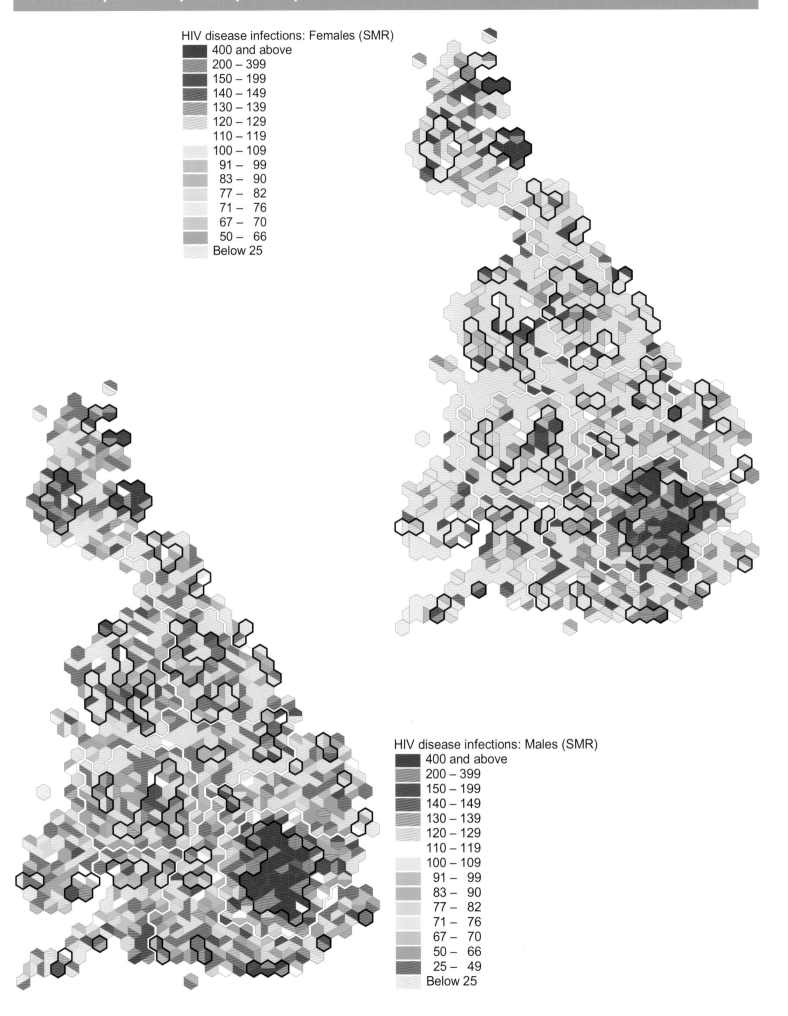

HIV disease infections: Females (SMR)

■	400 and above
	200 – 399
	150 – 199
	140 – 149
	130 – 139
	120 – 129
	110 – 119
	100 – 109
	91 – 99
	83 – 90
	77 – 82
	71 – 76
	67 – 70
	50 – 66
	Below 25

HIV disease infections: Males (SMR)

■	400 and above
	200 – 399
	150 – 199
	140 – 149
	130 – 139
	120 – 129
	110 – 119
	100 – 109
	91 – 99
	83 – 90
	77 – 82
	71 – 76
	67 – 70
	50 – 66
	25 – 49
	Below 25

29 AIR ACCIDENTS

This is a sub-category of deaths due to external causes (Map 5) and includes deaths from powered and unpowered aircraft (for example, gliders, hot air balloons).

900 cases

0.01% of all deaths

average age = 39.8

male:female ratio = 88:12

Note that we are mapping where people were living at the time of their death, not their actual location of death. The cluster of high SMRs in the north of Scotland reflects the use of small aircraft to travel between remote places and islands. Almost nine out of ten of these deaths are of males, probably reflecting the fact that men vastly outnumber women as both civilian and military pilots.

Air accidents are a very rare cause of death, but because air crashes often have dramatic outcomes, when they do occur they garner a lot of attention. Take-off and landing are the times when air accidents are most likely to occur. The majority of aircraft accidents are of private planes and helicopters.

In the UK the Air Accidents Investigation Branch, an independent part of the Department for Transport, investigates all civilian air crashes.

Although the amount of air traffic has been expanding in recent years, the number of air accidents fell to an all-time low in 2007 (*The Times*, 3 January 2008). Europe is the safest continent for air travel. The well-known maxim that flying is the safest form of transport for travelling long distances is indeed correct.

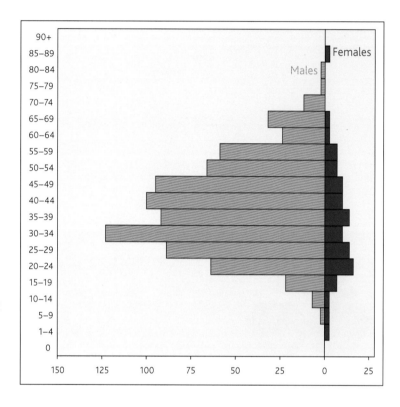

Thomas Selfridge was the first person to die in an air accident, in Virginia, USA, in 1908. Orville Wright survived the crash.

ICD-9 codes: E840-E844
ICD-10 codes: V95-V97

ICD-9	ICD-9 name	% of cases	ICD-10	ICD-10 name	% of cases
E840	Accident to powered aircraft at takeoff or landing	9.8	V95	Accident to powered aircraft causing injury to occupant	58.4
E841	Accident to powered aircraft, other and unspecified	67.2			
E842	Accident to unpowered aircraft	13.9	V96	Accident to non-powered aircraft causing injury to occupant	16.9
E844	Other specified air transport accidents	8.5	V97.2	Parachutist injured in air transport accident	18.2
	Other causes in group	0.6		Other causes in group	6.5
		100.0			100.0

MAP 29   AIR ACCIDENTS

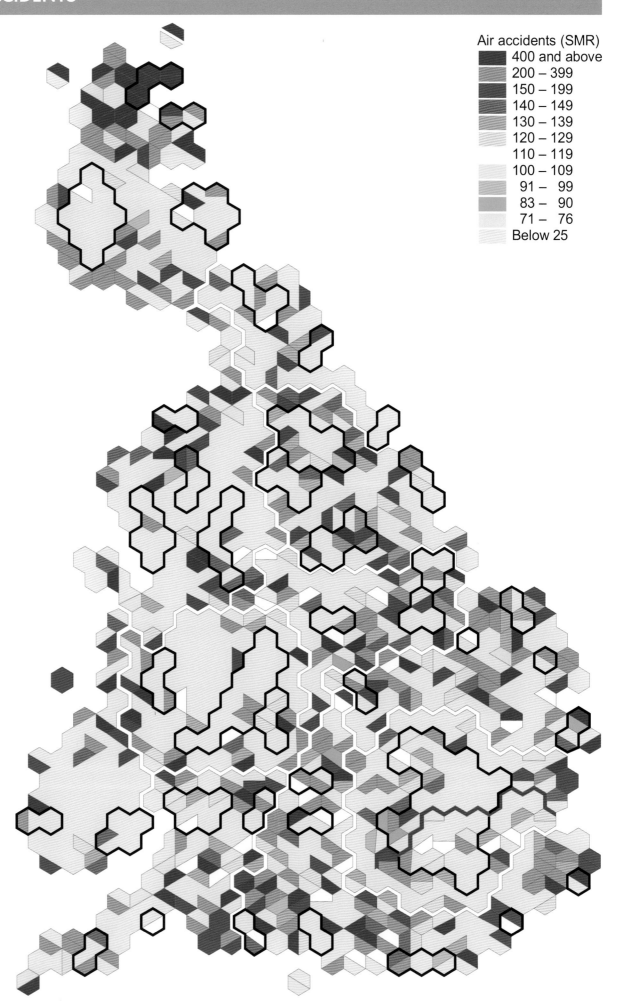

Air accidents (SMR)
- 400 and above
- 200 – 399
- 150 – 199
- 140 – 149
- 130 – 139
- 120 – 129
- 110 – 119
- 100 – 109
- 91 – 99
- 83 – 90
- 71 – 76
- Below 25

30 DEATHS CAUSED BY MACHINERY

This is a sub-category of deaths due to external causes (Map 5) and is a form of unintentional injury.

1,687 cases

0.01% of all deaths

average age = 40.4

male:female ratio = 97:3

These deaths are almost all of males with just 3% being of females and hence the map reflects the pattern for males. The SMRs tend to be highest in agricultural and industrial areas.

Most of the males who die from this cause are of working age (as seen in the age–sex bar chart). This reflects the fact that most such deaths are associated with occupations that involve using heavy machinery and these types of jobs are staffed almost exclusively by male workers. Examples of the types of machinery that can cause fatal injuries are drilling machines (for example, for building tunnels), threshing machines and baling machines (recycling plants are a recent and expanding site of such hazards).

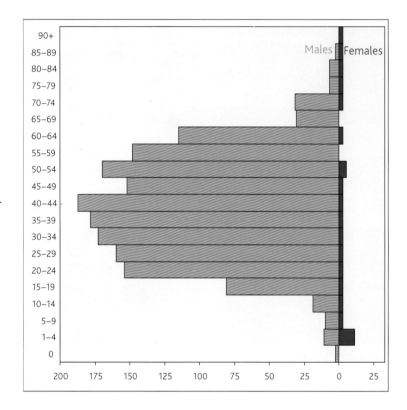

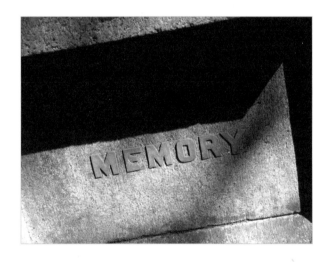

Often the death occurs when someone is attempting to repair the machine without correctly switching off the power source.

The Health and Safety Commission is responsible for protecting people's health and safety by ensuring risks in the changing workplace are properly controlled.

ICD-9 codes: E919
ICD-10 codes: W24, W30-W31

ICD-9	ICD-9 name	% of cases	ICD-10	ICD-10 name	% of cases
E919	Deaths caused by machinery	100.0	W24	Contact with lifting and transmission devices, not elsewhere classified	16.4
			W30	Contact with agricultural machinery	25.4
			W31	Contact with other and unspecified machinery	58.2
		100.0			100.0

MAP 30 DEATHS CAUSED BY MACHINERY.

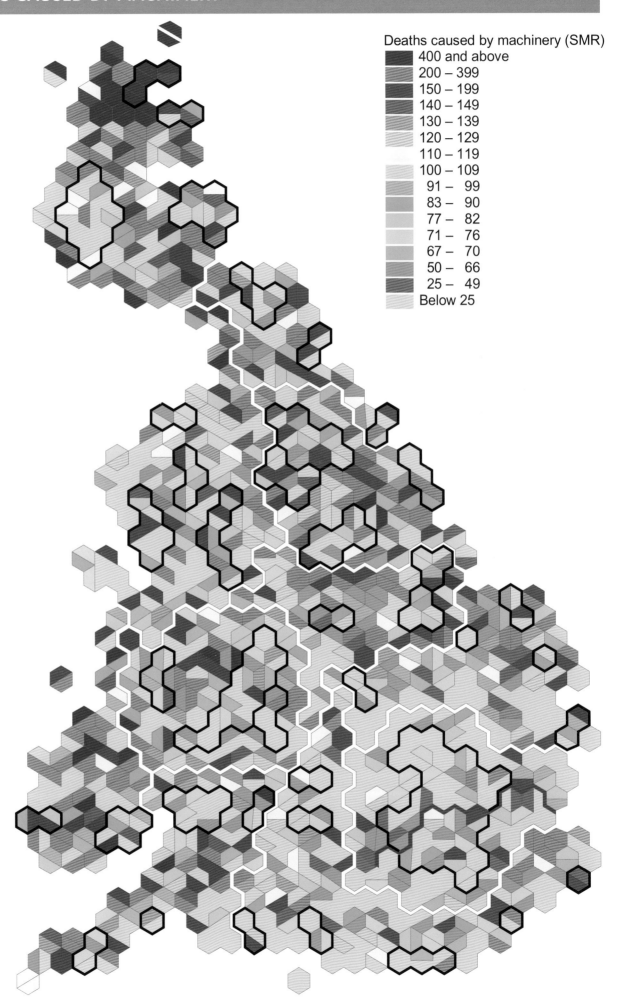

Deaths caused by machinery (SMR)

- 400 and above
- 200 – 399
- 150 – 199
- 140 – 149
- 130 – 139
- 120 – 129
- 110 – 119
- 100 – 109
- 91 – 99
- 83 – 90
- 77 – 82
- 71 – 76
- 67 – 70
- 50 – 66
- 25 – 49
- Below 25

31 OTHER SUICIDE/UNDETERMINED ACCIDENTS

This is a residual sub-category of deaths due to external causes and includes methods of suicide or accidents that are not included elsewhere. This includes: intentionally crashing a vehicle, jumping or lying before a moving object, and other events where the intent is not determined, but suicide is often a possibility.

27,288 cases

0.18% of all deaths

average age = 41.8

male:female ratio = 70:30

There is a female cluster of high SMRs in Inner London; for males there is an additional cluster in Manchester. The age–sex bar chart shows the predominance of male deaths and a distinct pattern by age group.

It is often difficult for a coroner to determine whether a death was suicide or an accident, which is why we have considered the two as one category.

The method of suicide that an individual chooses will be constrained by availability. Unless one has access to a firearm one cannot commit suicide by that method; a mobility-impaired person is perhaps unlikely to choose to jump to their death.

For the deaths of young children included here, infanticide, manslaughter or murder are likely to be possible explanations, rather than suicide. In general, a very small proportion of undetermined accidents will have been the result of murder, manslaughter, or other foul play.

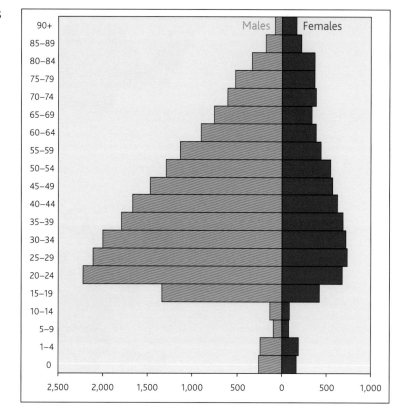

ICD-9 codes: E958-E959, E988-E989

ICD-10 codes: X76-X77, X81-X84, Y26-Y27, Y29, Y31, Y33-Y34, Y87.0, Y87.2

ICD-9	ICD-9 name	% of cases	ICD-10	ICD-10 name	% of cases
E958	Suicide and self-inflicted injury by other and unspecified means	30.7	X81	Intentional self-harm by jumping or lying before moving object	11.9
			X84	Intentional self-harm by unspecified means	8.9
E988	Injury by other and unspecified means, undetermined whether accidentally or purposely inflicted	69.0	Y33	Other specified events, undetermined intent	51.3
			Y34	Unspecified event, undetermined intent	14.1
	Other causes in group	0.3		Other causes in group	13.8
		100.0			100.0

MAP 31A (FEMALES) 31B (MALES)   OTHER SUICIDE/UNDETERMINED ACCIDENTS

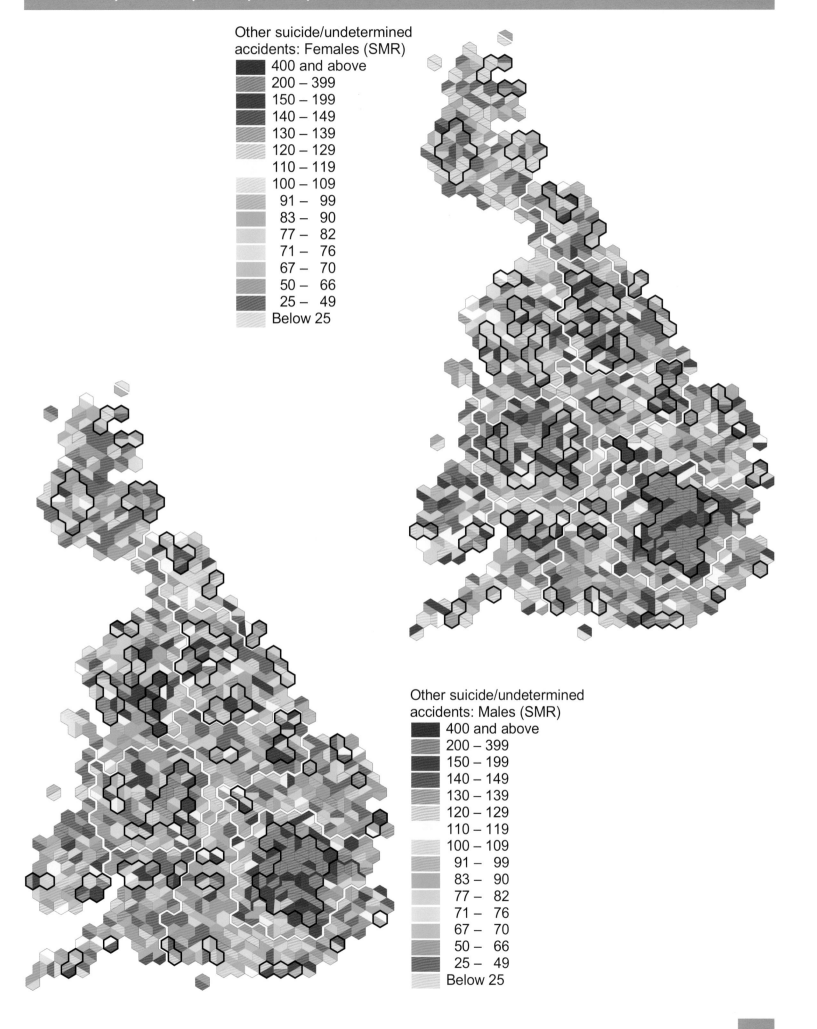

Other suicide/undetermined
accidents: Females (SMR)

	400 and above
	200 – 399
	150 – 199
	140 – 149
	130 – 139
	120 – 129
	110 – 119
	100 – 109
	91 – 99
	83 – 90
	77 – 82
	71 – 76
	67 – 70
	50 – 66
	25 – 49
	Below 25

Other suicide/undetermined
accidents: Males (SMR)

	400 and above
	200 – 399
	150 – 199
	140 – 149
	130 – 139
	120 – 129
	110 – 119
	100 – 109
	91 – 99
	83 – 90
	77 – 82
	71 – 76
	67 – 70
	50 – 66
	25 – 49
	Below 25

32 SUICIDE/UNDETERMINED BY GASES

This is a sub-category of deaths due to suicide, and relates to self-poisoning by exposure to gases and vapours, including carbon monoxide and motor vehicle exhaust gas. It also includes cases where intent is undetermined but suicide is often a possibility.

21,083 cases

0.14% of all deaths

average age = 41.9

male:female ratio = 89:11

The rates are noticeably low for this method of suicide in areas where many people do not own cars, such as in London. The rates are higher where households own several cars — and where more people have garages.

A common method of suicide that falls into this category is self-asphyxiation using car exhaust fumes. This is a method of suicide traditionally favoured by young and middle-aged males (Amos et al, 2001) and is duly reflected in the age–sex bar chart. The introduction of catalytic converters (that remove carbon monoxide) to cars in the 1990s had the effect of reducing the number of deaths from this cause. However, Amos et al (2001) reported evidence of a compensatory rise in rates of hanging among young and middle-aged men (see Map 34).

Similarly, when the domestic gas supply was switched from coal gas to natural gas (which does not contain carbon monoxide) there was a significant drop in the suicide rate using this method. That change occurred before the data that are shown here were collated.

Amos, T., Appleby, L. and K. Kiernan (2001) 'Changes in rates of suicide by car exhaust asphyxiation in England and Wales', *Psychological Medicine*, no 31, pp 935-9.

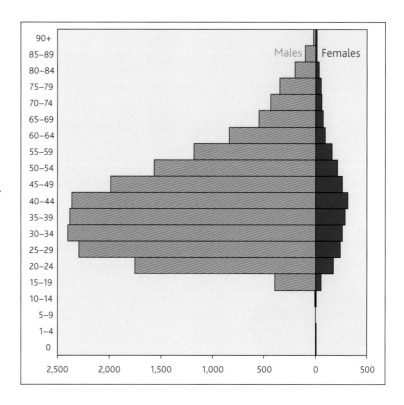

Poet Sylvia Plath and pathologist Sir Bernard Silsbury died from this cause.

ICD-9 codes: E951-E952, E981-E982
ICD-10 codes: X67, Y17

ICD-9	ICD-9 name	% of cases	ICD-10	ICD-10 name	% of cases
E952	Suicide and self-inflicted poisoning by other gases and vapours	91.5	X67	Intentional self-poisoning by and exposure to other gases and vapours	92.9
E982	Poisoning by other gases, undetermined whether accidentally or purposely inflicted	7.6	Y17	Poisoning by and exposure to other gases and vapours, undetermined intent	7.1
	Other causes in group	0.9			
		100.0			100.0

MAP 32A (FEMALES) 32B (MALES)   SUICIDE/UNDETERMINED BY GASES

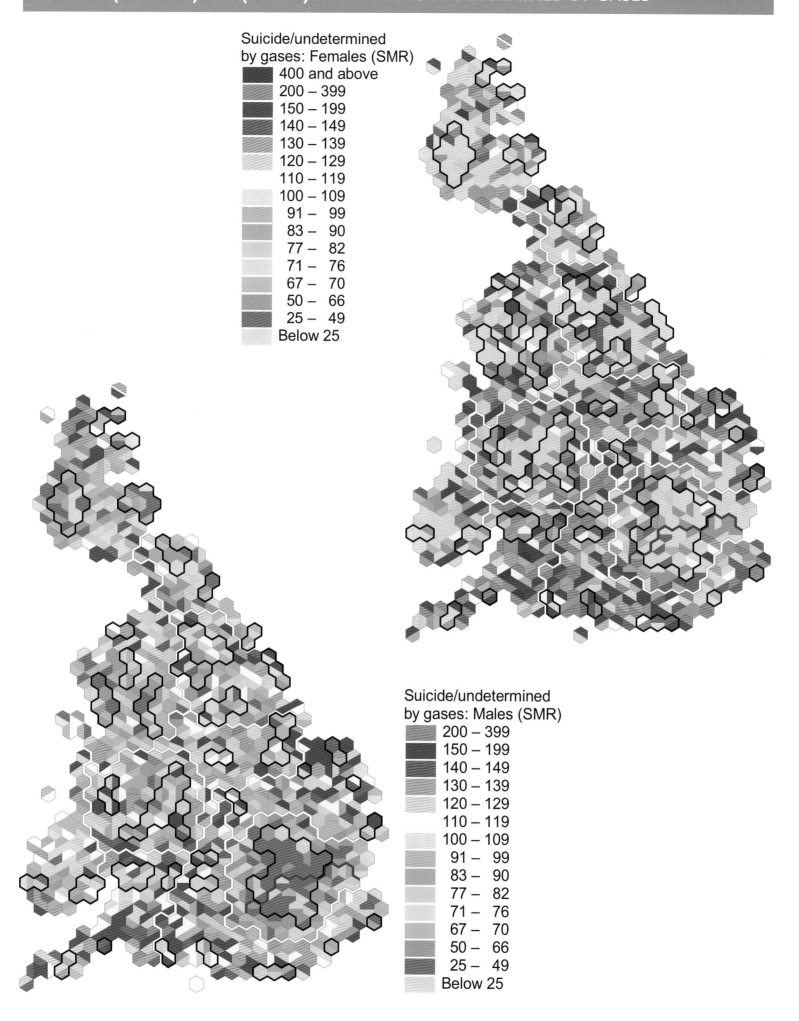

Suicide/undetermined
by gases: Females (SMR)

- 400 and above
- 200 – 399
- 150 – 199
- 140 – 149
- 130 – 139
- 120 – 129
- 110 – 119
- 100 – 109
- 91 – 99
- 83 – 90
- 77 – 82
- 71 – 76
- 67 – 70
- 50 – 66
- 25 – 49
- Below 25

Suicide/undetermined
by gases: Males (SMR)

- 200 – 399
- 150 – 199
- 140 – 149
- 130 – 139
- 120 – 129
- 110 – 119
- 100 – 109
- 91 – 99
- 83 – 90
- 77 – 82
- 71 – 76
- 67 – 70
- 50 – 66
- 25 – 49
- Below 25

34 SUICIDE/UNDETERMINED BY HANGING

This is a sub-category of deaths due to suicide and includes all intentional and undetermined deaths by means of hanging, as well as strangulation and suffocation.

41,861 cases

0.28% of all deaths

average age = 45.2

male:female ratio = 81:19

For both males and females, Edinburgh and Glasgow have the highest SMRs, followed by London.

Hanging is one of the most commonly used methods of suicide and its incidence has increased in the last 30 years, particularly among males under the age of 65 (Gunnell et al, 2005). This may possibly be explained in part by the substitution of hanging in place of other methods, such as gassing (see Map 32), which have become less prevalent in recent years.

The most commonly used ligatures are ropes, belts and electric flex, and the most commonly used ligature points are beams, banisters, hooks, door knobs and trees. In around half of cases the person is not fully suspended – the ligature point is below head level (for example, sitting on the floor and using a door knob).

Nine out of ten hangings occur in the community, the other 10% inside institutions such as prisons or hospitals. About seven out of ten of those who attempt to hang themselves are successful; the majority of those who reach hospital alive survive (Gunnell et al, 2005). Those who survive hanging may be left with severe neurological problems.

Among older females, suicide by means of suffocation using a plastic bag accounts for around a third of deaths in this category, as deaths by asphyxiation are included here.

Prevention of suicide by this method is difficult due to the widespread availability of ligatures and ligature points in the community.

Men who are in prison are five times more likely to commit suicide than men in the general population and prison suicide rates have been increasing over the past quarter of a century (Fazel et al, 2005).

Fazel, S., Benning, R. and Danesh, J. (2005) 'Suicides in male prisoners in England and Wales, 1978-2003', *Lancet*, no 366, pp 1301-2.

Gunnell, D., Benewith, O., Hawton, K., Simkin, S. and Kapur, N. (2005) 'The epidemiology and prevention of suicide by hanging: a systematic review', *International Journal of Epidemiology*, vol 34, no 2, pp 433-42.

Ian Curtis of Joy Division hanged himself in 1980. Convicted murderers Harold Shipman and Fred West hanged themselves while in prison.

ICD-9 codes: E953, E983
ICD-10 codes: X70, Y20

ICD-9	ICD-9 name	% of cases	ICD-10	ICD-10 name	% of cases
E953	Suicide and self-inflicted injury by hanging, strangulation and suffocation	89.0	X70	Intentional self-harm by hanging, strangulation and suffocation	87.3
E983	Hanging, strangulation or suffocation, undetermined whether accidentally or purposely inflicted	11.0	Y20	Hanging, strangulation and suffocation, undetermined intent	12.7
		100.0			100.0

MAP 34A (FEMALES) 34B (MALES)   SUICIDE/UNDETERMINED BY HANGING

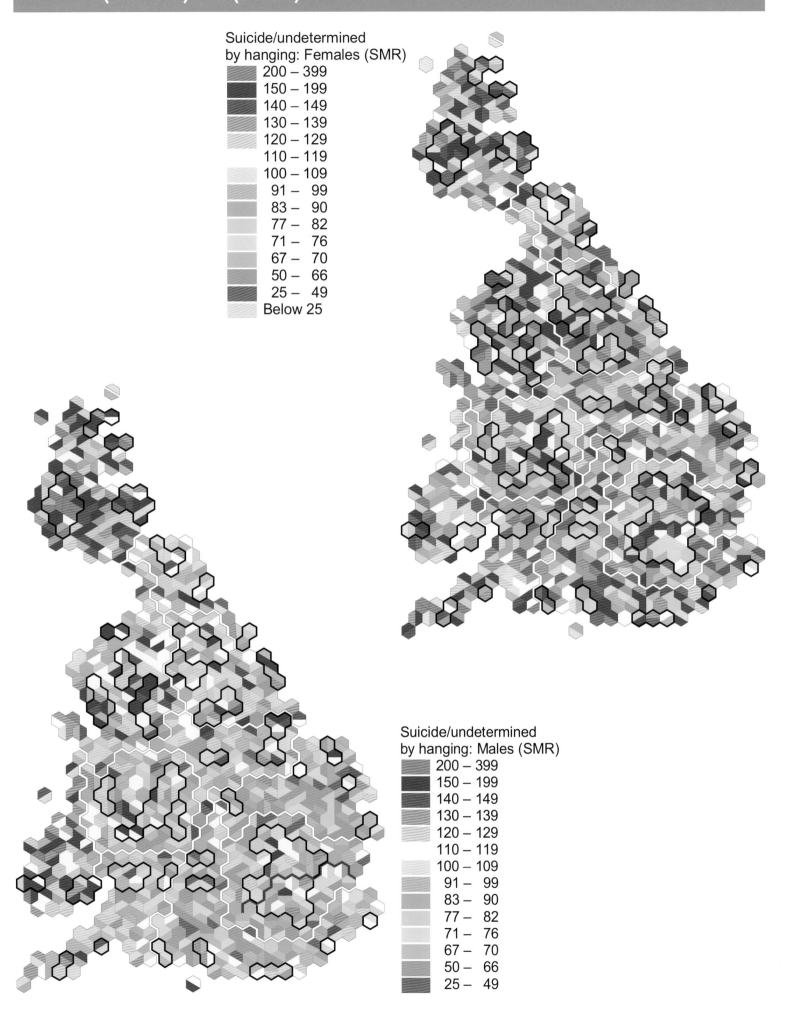

Suicide/undetermined
by hanging: Females (SMR)
- 200 – 399
- 150 – 199
- 140 – 149
- 130 – 139
- 120 – 129
- 110 – 119
- 100 – 109
- 91 – 99
- 83 – 90
- 77 – 82
- 71 – 76
- 67 – 70
- 50 – 66
- 25 – 49
- Below 25

Suicide/undetermined
by hanging: Males (SMR)
- 200 – 399
- 150 – 199
- 140 – 149
- 130 – 139
- 120 – 129
- 110 – 119
- 100 – 109
- 91 – 99
- 83 – 90
- 77 – 82
- 71 – 76
- 67 – 70
- 50 – 66
- 25 – 49

35 SUICIDE/UNDETERMINED BY FIREARMS

This is a sub-category of deaths due to suicide and includes all intentional deaths by means of firearms as well as those where the intent was undetermined, but suicide was a possibility.

See also Map 20 Assault using firearms.

4,619 cases

0.03% of all deaths

average age = 46.4

male:female ratio = 95:5

As with the other categories of death related to suicide shown here, many of the undetermined cases may have been actual suicide attempts, but without conclusive evidence such as an authentic suicide note. Alternatively, the death may have been truly accidental. In only one eighth of the cases under ICD-9 was a possibility of accident reflected in the cause recorded on death certification. That proportion has risen slightly in more recent years.

Only one in 20 of these deaths are of females, a pattern starkly illustrated in the age–sex bar chart. The map therefore effectively reflects the rate for males.

In terms of prevention, the rate of suicide (and also homicide) using firearms has been found to be related to access to firearms and the availability of firearms within the home. The safer storage of firearms – keeping them locked and unloaded – within the home can reduce the likelihood that they will be used as an impulsive method of suicide.

Another facet of access to suicide methods is occupation. The occupations with the highest rates of suicide using firearms are farmers, forestry workers, veterinarians and farm workers.

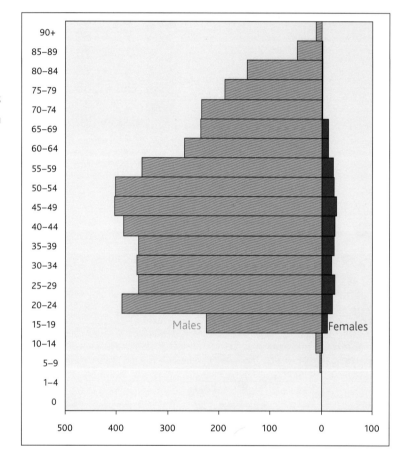

Singer-songwriter Kurt Cobain, author Ernest Hemingway and journalist Hunter S. Thompson died from this cause.

ICD-9 codes: E955, E985
ICD-10 codes: X72-X75, Y22-Y24

ICD-9	ICD-9 name	% of cases	ICD-10	ICD-10 name	% of cases
E955	Suicide and self-inflicted injury by firearms and explosives	87.2	X73	Intentional self-harm by rifle, shotgun and larger firearm discharge	43.4
			X74	Intentional self-harm by other and unspecified firearm discharge	40.2
E985	Injury by firearms and explosives, undetermined whether accidentally or purposely inflicted	12.8	Y23	Rifle, shotgun and larger firearm discharge, undetermined intent	7.4
			Y24	Other and unspecified firearm discharge, undetermined intent	6.7
				Other causes in group	2.3
		100.0			100.0

MAP 35   SUICIDE/UNDETERMINED BY FIREARMS

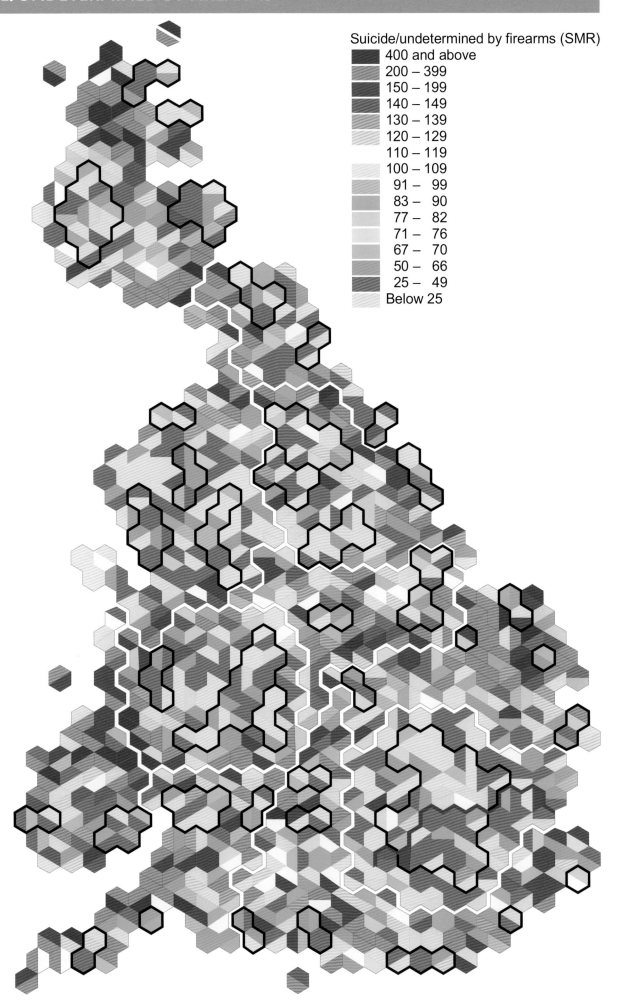

Suicide/undetermined by firearms (SMR)

- 400 and above
- 200 – 399
- 150 – 199
- 140 – 149
- 130 – 139
- 120 – 129
- 110 – 119
- 100 – 109
- 91 – 99
- 83 – 90
- 77 – 82
- 71 – 76
- 67 – 70
- 50 – 66
- 25 – 49
- Below 25

36 ACCIDENTAL POISONING

This is a sub-category of external deaths and includes accidental poisoning by a chemical, noxious substance, gas or vapour.

See also Map 38 Suicide/undetermined by poison.

3,546 cases

0.02% of all deaths

average age = 48.1

male:female ratio = 72:28

Nearly three quarters of deaths in this category are of males. Rates tend to be higher on the western side of Britain. Rates are somewhat higher in poorer and colder areas more likely to have faulty boilers in use.

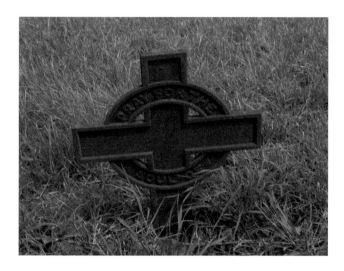

These are deaths that the coroner has judged to be genuine accidents. They might include such deaths as accidental overdoses, perhaps by misinterpreting the advice for taking a prescription or by taking the drugs prescribed for someone else.

Many of the deaths in this category are due to carbon monoxide poisoning. Carbon monoxide can be produced by faulty home fuel-burning heating equipment, most usually boilers. It is colourless, odourless and tasteless, making it difficult for people to detect. Symptoms of mild poisoning include headaches, depression, flu-like symptoms and vertigo. Deaths can be prevented by correct installation and the regular servicing of equipment and by using carbon monoxide detectors.

It is estimated that 20,000 people died due to the Bhopal disaster when 40 tonnes of pesticide were released into the heart of the city of Bhopal in India in 1984.

ICD-9 codes: E861-E869
ICD-10 codes: X47-X49

ICD-9	ICD-9 name	% of cases	ICD-10	ICD-10 name	% of cases
E862	Accidental poisoning by petroleum products, other solvents and their vapours, not elsewhere classified	6.0			
E866	Accidental poisoning by other and unspecified solid and liquid substances	5.3	X49	Accidental poisoning by and exposure to other and unspecified chemicals and noxious substances	39.1
E867	Accidental poisoning by gas distributed by pipeline	17.0			
E868	Accidental poisoning by other utility gas and other carbon monoxide	56.4			
E869	Accidental poisoning by other gases and vapours	9.9	X47	Accidental poisoning by and exposure to other gases and vapours	59.2
	Other causes in group	5.4		Other causes in group	1.7
		100.0			100.0

MAP 36   ACCIDENTAL POISONING

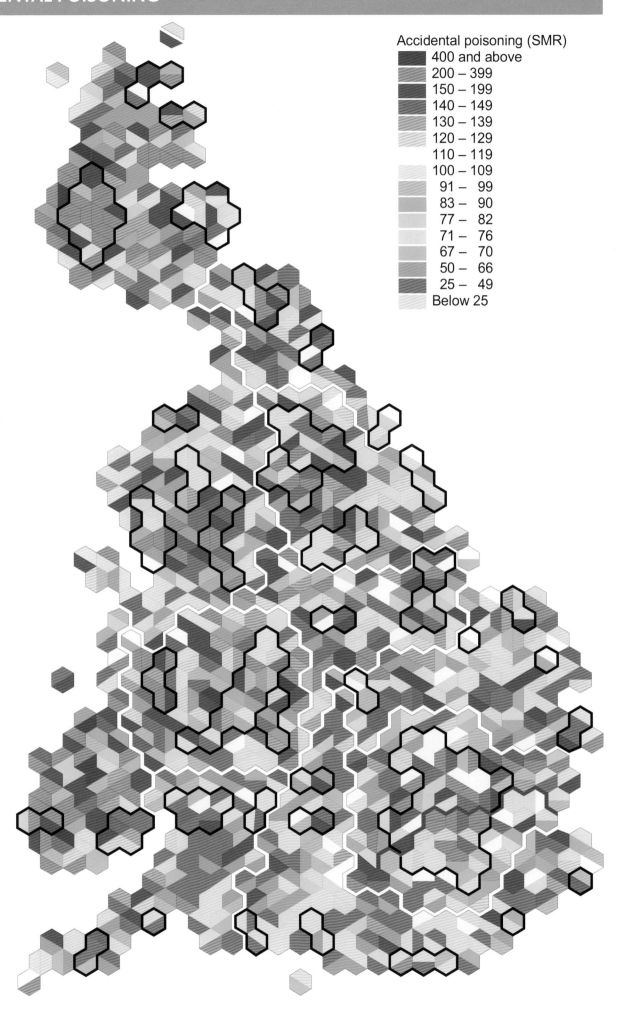

Accidental poisoning (SMR)

- 400 and above
- 200 – 399
- 150 – 199
- 140 – 149
- 130 – 139
- 120 – 129
- 110 – 119
- 100 – 109
- 91 – 99
- 83 – 90
- 77 – 82
- 71 – 76
- 67 – 70
- 50 – 66
- 25 – 49
- Below 25

37   EPILEPSY

Epilepsy is a chronic neurological condition characterised by recurrent seizures that cannot be attributed to any other cause. It is the most common chronic neurological condition in the UK.

21,991 cases

0.15% of all deaths

average age = 48.3

male:female ratio = 57:43

There is very possibly an observable association with deprivation/poor management as shown in the maps here. If this were the case then epilepsy could for some purposes be grouped with other causes for which deaths are exacerbated due to low rates of early diagnosis, or poor subsequent management for poorer social groups clustered in certain areas. At the same time, it is very possible that selective migration of people suffering from severe epilepsy leads to geographic concentrations of the population most at risk.

Epilepsy is considered to be a cause of death that is amenable to medical treatment. Not all deaths that are amenable to treatment will be avoidable, but health care could contribute to reducing mortality from that cause. Variations in the treatment and management of epilepsy may help to explain any variations observed here.

If a person has two or more seizures for which no other reason is found, they are probably epileptic. Seizures can occur at any time and may stop and start for no apparent reason.

A seizure is essentially abnormal electrical activity of a group of brain cells which can lead to an altered mental state, convulsions and involuntary muscle movements. The symptoms experienced reflect the area of the brain that is affected. In some cases the full onset of a seizure may be preceded by warning sensations such as smelling an unpleasant odour or seeing sparkling or flashes; this is called an 'aura'.

A number of social, psychological and emotional problems can often accompany the condition of epilepsy. The stigma of being marked out as different, the unpredictability of the seizures, and the nature of seizures can all have significant effects on how a person is able to cope with their disease. The unpleasant side effects of medication, having to limit certain activities, and not being able to drive can lead to social isolation and low self-esteem. Epileptics have a higher risk of suicide than non-epileptics (Bruce et al, 2004).

Bruce, M., Griffiths, C. and Brock, A. (2004) 'Trends in mortality and hospital related admissions associated with epilepsy in England and Wales during the 1990s', *Health Statistics Quarterly*, no 21, pp 23-9.

Notable epileptics: writer and artist Edward Lear, musician Neil Young, singer Ian Curtis and athlete Florence Griffith Joyner (Flo Jo).

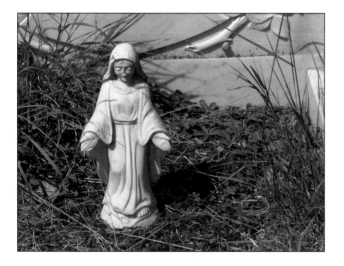

ICD-9 codes: 345
ICD-10 codes: G40-G41

ICD-9	ICD-9 name	% of cases	ICD-10	ICD-10 name	% of cases
345	Epilepsy	100.0	G40	Epilepsy	91.4
			G41	Status epilepticus	8.6
		100.0			100.0

MAP 37   EPILEPSY

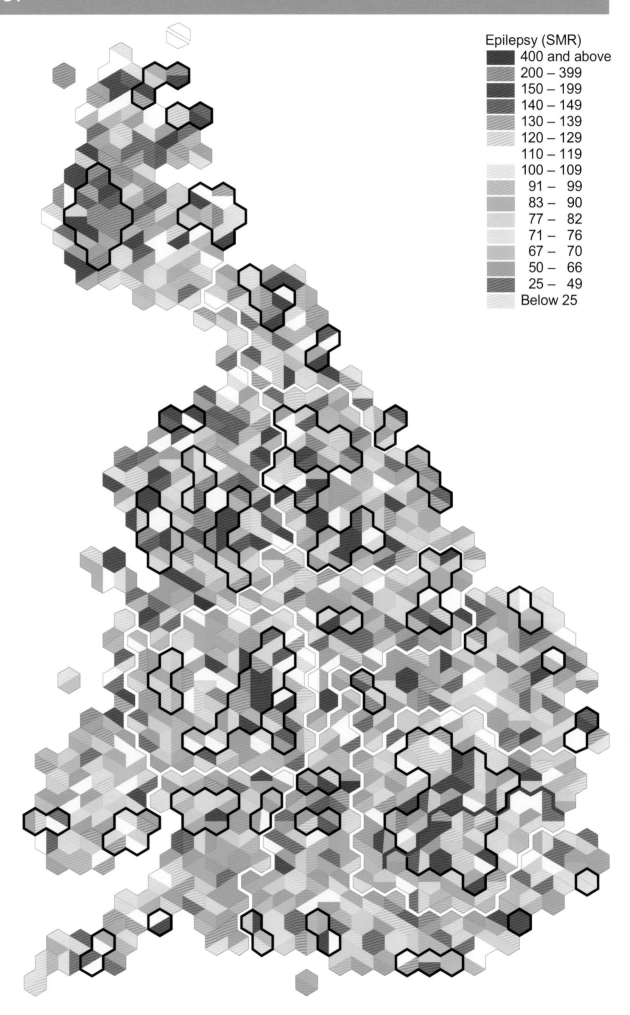

Epilepsy (SMR)

	400 and above
	200 – 399
	150 – 199
	140 – 149
	130 – 139
	120 – 129
	110 – 119
	100 – 109
	91 – 99
	83 – 90
	77 – 82
	71 – 76
	67 – 70
	50 – 66
	25 – 49
	Below 25

38 SUICIDE/UNDETERMINED BY POISON

This category includes deaths due to poisoning that a coroner has determined as suicides, and those where the individual's intent remains undetermined, although many such cases are likely to be (unproven) suicide.

See also Map 19 Deaths due to drugs.

40,830 cases

0.28% of all deaths

average age = 48.4

male:female ratio = 51:49

As with many other causes of death, Scotland, and Glasgow in particular, has the highest SMRs. Further clusters are found in Brighton, Manchester and south London, the remainder of the country showing a north–south divide.

This category includes people who have taken their lives, intentionally or with undetermined intent, by ingesting drugs or other poisons of some kind. This might include over-the-counter drugs such as paracetamol, or illegal drugs such as heroin, and other chemicals such as pesticides and household chemicals.

These deaths are evenly distributed among males and females in terms of total numbers (51% and 49% respectively) although the age distributions are different, with more males dying of this cause at a younger age. Rates from this one group of causes peaked at ages 35–39 for men and at 50–54 for women over the period as a whole.

Alan Turing, a mathematician and code-breaker who worked at Bletchley Park during the Second World War, and Cleopatra (69 BC–30 BC) died from this cause.

ICD-9 codes: E950, E980
ICD-10 codes: X60-X66, X68-X69, Y10-Y16, Y18-Y19

ICD-9	ICD-9 name	% of cases	ICD-10	ICD-10 name	% of cases
E950	Suicide and self-inflicted poisoning by solid or liquid substances	62.9	X60	Intentional self-poisoning by and exposure to nonopioid analgesics, antipyretics and antirheumatics	6.3
			X61	Intentional self-poisoning by and exposure to antiepileptic, sedative-hypnotic, anti-Parkinsonism and psychotropic drugs, not elsewhere classified	16.6
			X62	Intentional self-poisoning by and exposure to narcotics and psychodysleptics [hallucinogens], not elsewhere classified	10.8
			X64	Intentional self-poisoning by and exposure to other and unspecified drugs, medicaments and biological substances	20.9
E980	Poisoning by solid or liquid substances, undetermined whether accidentally or purposely inflicted	37.1	Y11	Poisoning by and exposure to antiepileptic, sedative-hypnotic, anti-Parkinsonism and psychotropic drugs, not elsewhere classified, undetermined intent	11.4
			Y12	Poisoning by and exposure to narcotics and psychodysleptics [hallucinogens], not elsewhere classified, undetermined intent	11.8
			Y14	Poisoning by and exposure to other and unspecified drugs, medicaments and biological substances, undetermined intent	14.3
				Other causes in group	7.9
		100.0			100.0

MAP 38 SUICIDE/UNDETERMINED BY POISON

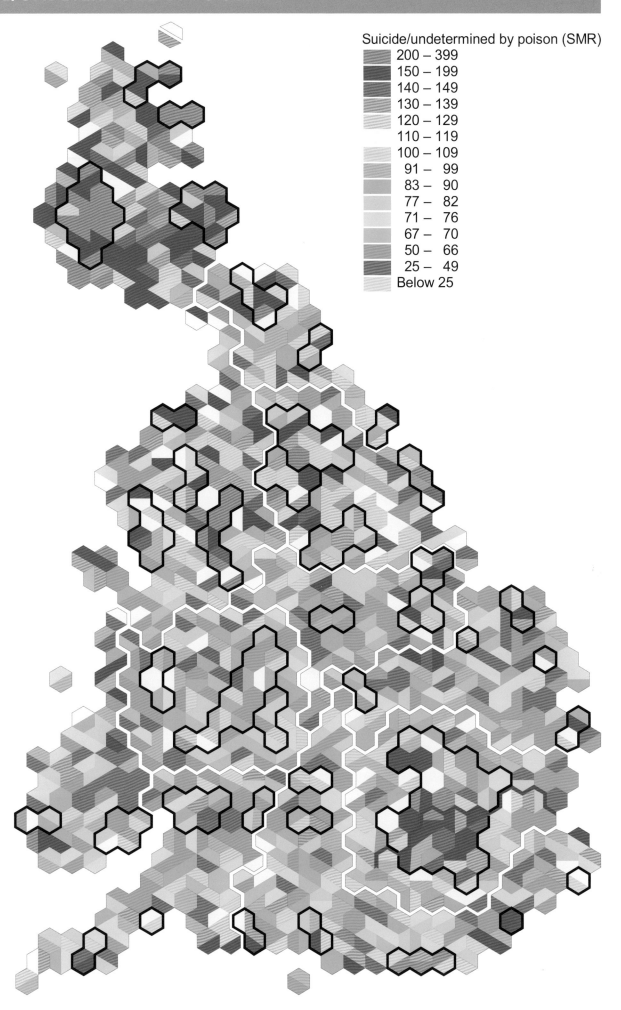

Suicide/undetermined by poison (SMR)

	200 – 399
	150 – 199
	140 – 149
	130 – 139
	120 – 129
	110 – 119
	100 – 109
	91 – 99
	83 – 90
	77 – 82
	71 – 76
	67 – 70
	50 – 66
	25 – 49
	Below 25

39 SUICIDE/UNDETERMINED BY CUTTING

This category includes deaths due to cutting that a coroner has determined as suicides, and those where the individual's intent remains undetermined, although many such cases are likely to be unproven suicide. The undetermined account for one sixth of the total deaths here.

See also Map 18 Assault by cutting.

2,612 cases

0.02% of all deaths

average age = 50.7

male:female ratio = 81:19

Four out of five deaths due to this cause are of males. The map reveals a cluster of high SMRs in Glasgow, followed by further clusters in London.

The deaths in this category are caused by cutting by using a sharp object such as a knife (often a domestic kitchen knife), razor, or broken glass. The location of the cut is often the arteries of the wrist or throat. This cutting causes *exsanguination*, or death by blood loss.

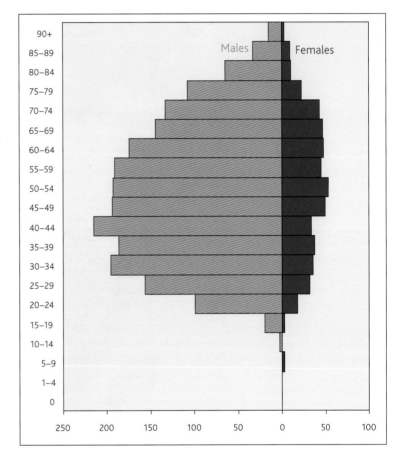

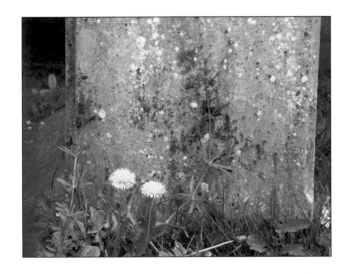

The age–sex bar chart illustrates the gender imbalance (81% of such deaths being of males), peaking for 30–65-year-old males; this method is not the preserve of the young or the old.

ICD-9 codes: E956, E986
ICD-10 codes: X78, Y28

ICD-9	ICD-9 name	% of cases	ICD-10	ICD-10 name	% of cases
E956	Suicide and self-inflicted injury by cutting and piercing instruments	85.5	X78	Intentional self-harm by sharp object	80.8
E986	Injury by cutting and piercing instruments, undetermined whether accidentally or purposely inflicted	14.5	Y28	Contact with sharp object, undetermined intent	19.2
		100.0			100.0

MAP 39 SUICIDE/UNDETERMINED BY CUTTING

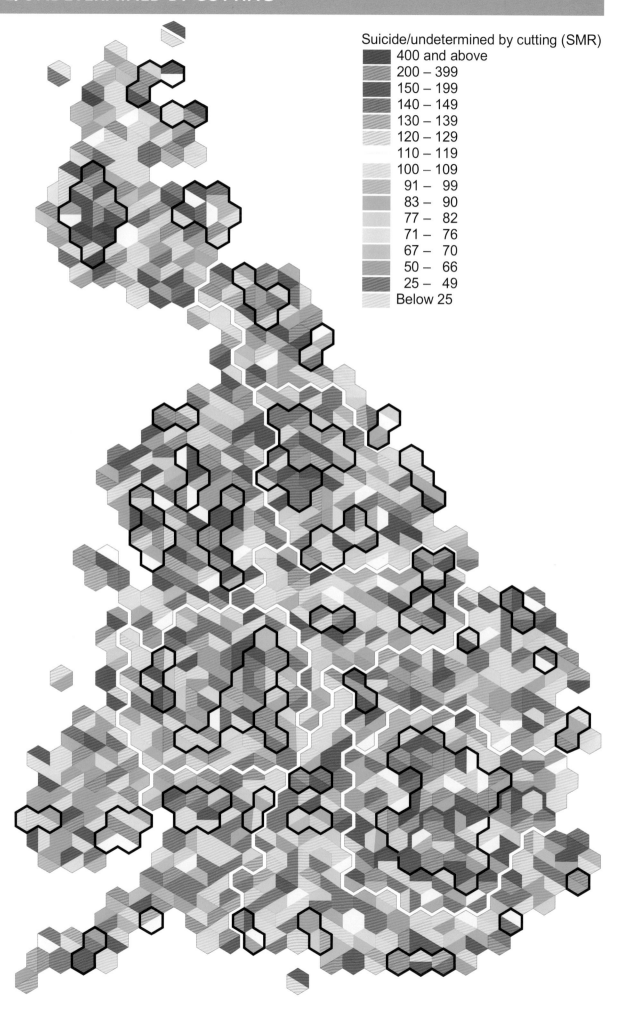

Suicide/undetermined by cutting (SMR)

- 400 and above
- 200 – 399
- 150 – 199
- 140 – 149
- 130 – 139
- 120 – 129
- 110 – 119
- 100 – 109
- 91 – 99
- 83 – 90
- 77 – 82
- 71 – 76
- 67 – 70
- 50 – 66
- 25 – 49
- Below 25

40   DUE TO ALCOHOL

This category includes deaths due to alcohol abuse, alcohol dependence and alcohol poisoning. Nearly half of deaths in this grouping were due to *alcohol dependence syndrome*. The popular term for alcohol dependence is *alcoholism*.

See also Map 47 Chronic liver disease.

16,982 cases

0.11% of all deaths

average age = 51.2

male:female ratio = 70:30

The geographical pattern for this cause of death is one of the most striking. A third of deaths due to this cause are in Scotland. Glasgow, Edinburgh, Dundee and the northernmost parts of Scotland have the highest SMRs. The divide between Scotland and England is sharp – with only one part of one northern city (Newcastle) having rates comparable to much of Scotland.

70% of deaths for this cause are of males; for both males and females deaths peak in the 45–55-year-old age group.

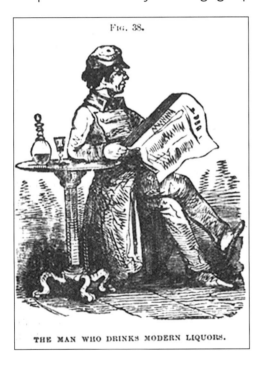

Fig. 38.

THE MAN WHO DRINKS MODERN LIQUORS.

Deaths from liver disease, many cancers, illegal drugs and suicide are not included here even when alcohol contributed to them.

Alcohol consumption patterns, whether within recommended 'safe' levels or in excess of these, are very much determined by the prevalent cultural and social values in a society. In Mediterranean countries alcohol is usually consumed with meals, and getting drunk is frowned upon. In the UK more people drink in order to get drunk, and being drunk is much more socially acceptable, and in some situations (for example, stag and hen parties) virtually demanded.

The ONS has produced a number of reports on alcohol-related deaths which include this and also other causes (for example, chronic liver disease and cirrhosis; alcoholic cardiomyopathy) but not accidents and assaults related to alcohol, suicides, or other causes of death to which alcohol may have a causal link for example, oesophageal cancer. The alcohol-related death rate in the UK almost doubled between 1991 and 2006 (ONS, 2008).

ONS (2008) *Alcohol-related death rates continue to rise*, News release, 25 January.

Some notable people who died due to alcohol problems are poet Dylan Thomas, artist Henri Toulouse-Lautrec, author Jack Kerouac and footballer George Best.

ICD-9 codes: 291, 303, 305.0, E860

ICD-10 codes: F10, F55, X45

ICD-9	ICD-9 name	% of cases	ICD-10	ICD-10 name	% of cases
303	Alcohol dependence syndrome	47.8	F10	Mental and behavioural disorders due to use of alcohol	86.7
305	Alcohol abuse	29.7			
E860	Accidental poisoning by alcohol, not elsewhere classified	19.7	X45	Accidental poisoning by and exposure to alcohol	13.0
	Other causes in group	2.8		Other causes in group	0.3
		100.0			100.0

MAP 40   DUE TO ALCOHOL

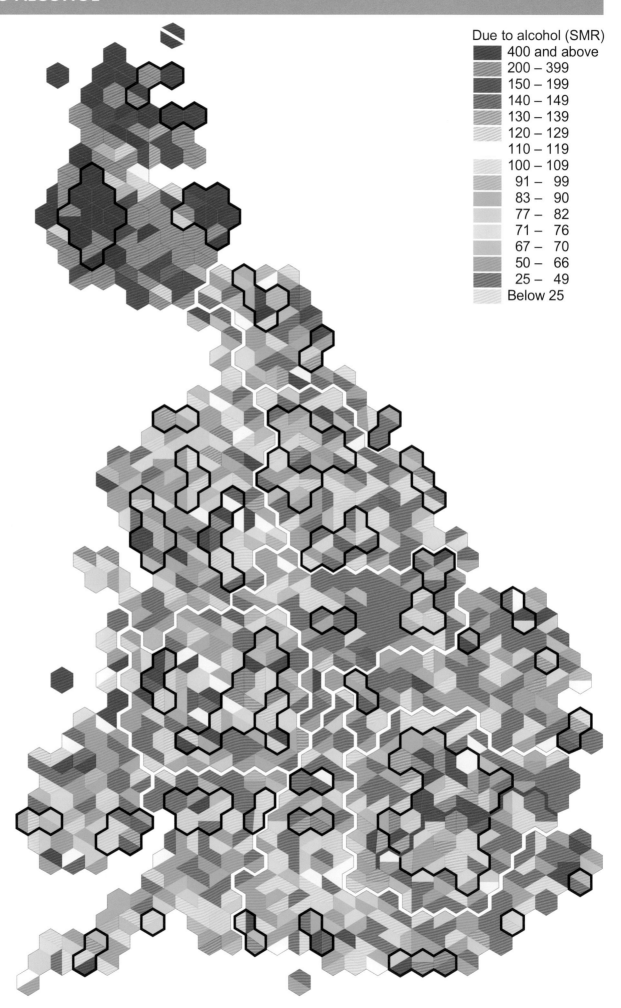

Due to alcohol (SMR)
- 400 and above
- 200 – 399
- 150 – 199
- 140 – 149
- 130 – 139
- 120 – 129
- 110 – 119
- 100 – 109
- 91 – 99
- 83 – 90
- 77 – 82
- 71 – 76
- 67 – 70
- 50 – 66
- 25 – 49
- Below 25

41   PEDESTRIAN HIT BY VEHICLE

This category includes deaths to pedestrians due to collision with a vehicle of some kind.

See also Map 25 Pedal cyclist hit by vehicle, and Map 22 Motor vehicle accidents, which covers the deaths of the occupants of motor vehicles and motorcyclists.

29,008 cases

0.20% of all deaths

average age = 51.8

male:female ratio = 61:39

The highest SMRs are found in urban areas, while rural south west England has the lowest rates. Contrast this with Map 22, which covers the deaths of those who are drivers or passengers: on that map, the highest SMRs are found in rural areas.

The age distribution for this cause of death is unusual in that for both men and women there are two peaks – in the teenage years/ early 20s and later in the 70s and 80s (see age–sex bar chart). The peak in the younger age group is likely to reflect activity patterns – going out a lot and perhaps also not observing the Green Cross Code of their childhood. The more children are sheltered from cars when they are young, the less experience they will have of dealing with them; there is a tendency to blame victims of the road for their early deaths. The peak for the older age groups indicates the vulnerability of older people – they can generally move less quickly and their bodies are more fragile and less likely to heal.

For each mile travelled there are nearly 30 times more child pedestrian deaths than there are deaths to child car occupants (Sonkin et al, 2006). The children who are more likely to be pedestrians are those from lower-income families who are less likely to have a car. Strategies to reduce the number of pedestrian deaths include education, 20mph speed limits and speed bumps.

Philosopher Roland Barthes died from this cause.

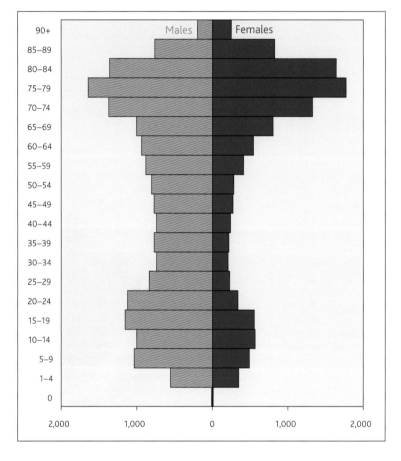

Sonkin, B., Edwards, P., Roberts, I. and Green, J. (2006) 'Walking, cycling and transport safety: an analysis of child road deaths', *Journal of the Royal Society of Medicine*, no 99, pp 402-5.

ICD-9 codes: E812.7, E813.7, E814.7, E815.7, E816.7, E817.7, E818.7, E819.7, E821.7, E822.7, E823.7, E824.7, E825.7, E826.0
ICD-10 codes: V01-V04, V06, V09.0-V09.3

ICD-9	ICD-9 name	% of cases	ICD-10	ICD-10 name	% of cases
E814.7	Motor vehicle traffic accident involving collision with pedestrian – Pedestrian	97.1	V03.1	Pedestrian injured in collision with car, pick-up truck or van – Traffic accident	49.0
			V04.1	Pedestrian injured in collision with heavy transport vehicle or bus – Traffic accident	17.1
			V09.2	Pedestrian injured in traffic accident involving other and unspecified motor vehicles	14.9
			V09.3	Pedestrian injured in unspecified traffic accident	9.7
	Other causes in group	2.9		Other causes in group	9.3
		100.0			100.0

MAP 41   PEDESTRIAN HIT BY VEHICLE

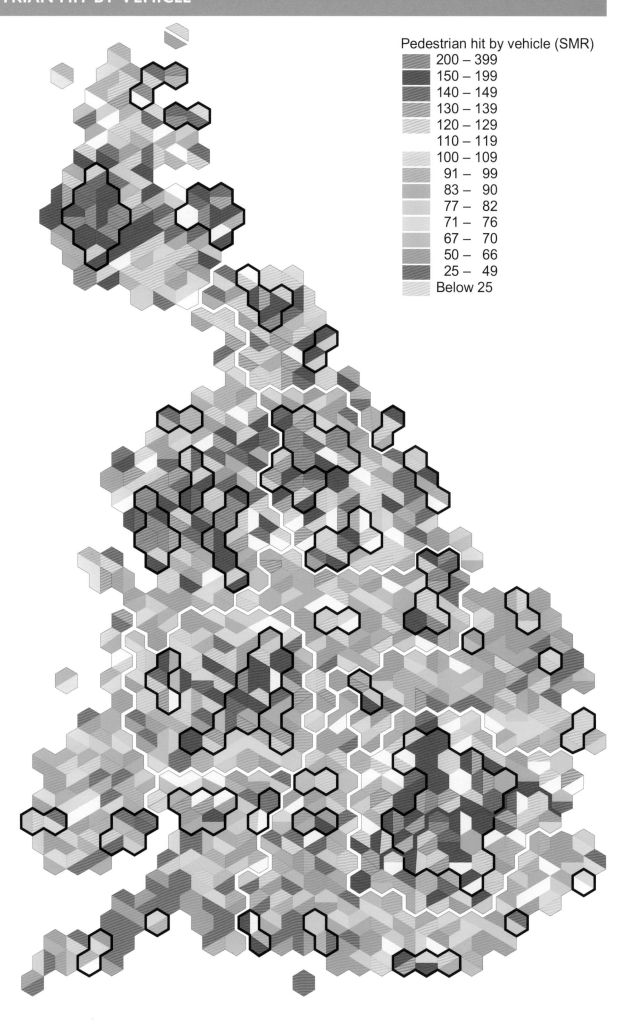

Pedestrian hit by vehicle (SMR)
- 200 – 399
- 150 – 199
- 140 – 149
- 130 – 139
- 120 – 129
- 110 – 119
- 100 – 109
- 91 – 99
- 83 – 90
- 77 – 82
- 71 – 76
- 67 – 70
- 50 – 66
- 25 – 49
- Below 25

42   SUICIDE/UNDETERMINED BY DROWNING

This category includes deaths due to drowning that a coroner has determined as suicides, and those where the individual's intent remains undetermined, although many such cases are likely to be unproven suicide.

See also Map 27 Accidental drowning.

12,175 cases

0.08% of all deaths

average age = 55.0

male:female ratio = 62:38

The highest SMRs for males and females are found in the north west of Scotland and in Glasgow, with a further cluster in London. Females also have high rates in Scotland but elsewhere the pattern is less evident. The lowest rates are most concentrated in a ring around outer London, mostly in the Home Counties.

This method of suicide accounts for less than one tenth (7.8%) of all suicides. However, it is a more common form of suicide for older people, particularly women, than for younger people. This is reflected in the mean age for this form of suicide – it has the highest mean age of all the categories of suicide.

Some of these deaths of older people may possibly be explained by cardiac arrest and subsequent drowning in the bath (which may be difficult to ascertain from a post-mortem) rather than due to deliberate suicide. The role of alcohol in these drowning deaths is unclear as death certificates do not contain sufficient data to explore this.

This method of suicide is not classed as amenable to specific prevention activities.

Of the specified suicide/undetermined causes, drowning has the highest proportion of undetermined deaths, with 63% being undetermined.

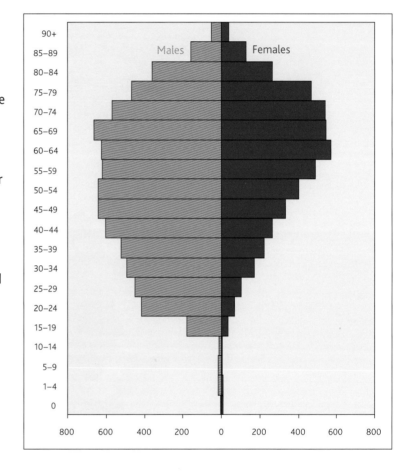

Novelist Virginia Woolf died from this cause.

ICD-9 codes: E954, E984
ICD-10 codes: X71, Y21

ICD-9	ICD-9 name	% of cases	ICD-10	ICD-10 name	% of cases
E954	Suicide and self-inflicted injury by submersion [drowning]	37.1	X71	Intentional self-harm by drowning and submersion	33.2
E984	Submersion [drowning], undetermined whether accidentally or purposely inflicted	62.9	Y21	Drowning and submersion, undetermined intent	66.8
		100.0			100.0

MAP 42A (FEMALES) 42B (MALES)　　SUICIDE/UNDETERMINED BY DROWNING

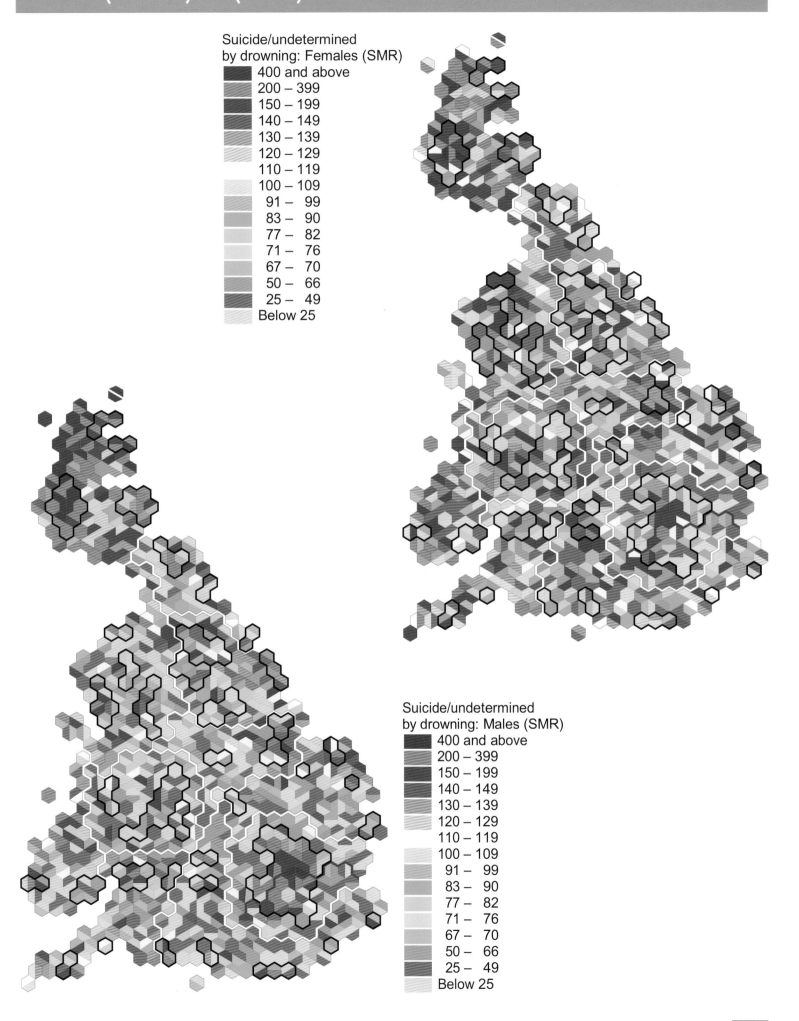

Suicide/undetermined
by drowning: Females (SMR)

- 400 and above
- 200 – 399
- 150 – 199
- 140 – 149
- 130 – 139
- 120 – 129
- 110 – 119
- 100 – 109
- 91 – 99
- 83 – 90
- 77 – 82
- 71 – 76
- 67 – 70
- 50 – 66
- 25 – 49
- Below 25

Suicide/undetermined
by drowning: Males (SMR)

- 400 and above
- 200 – 399
- 150 – 199
- 140 – 149
- 130 – 139
- 120 – 129
- 110 – 119
- 100 – 109
- 91 – 99
- 83 – 90
- 77 – 82
- 71 – 76
- 67 – 70
- 50 – 66
- 25 – 49
- Below 25

43 FIRE

This category includes deaths due to fire.

Many of those who die from this cause will die from burns, others from smoke inhalation.

14,095 cases

0.10% of all deaths

average age = 55.6

male:female ratio = 55:45

All of the neighbourhoods with SMRs of 400 and over are in Scotland, and of these, all bar two (Eilean Siar Rural and Hamilton North) are in Glasgow. Scotland is followed by London and then the more urban parts of the country with more high-rise buildings. In comparison, rural areas tend to have much lower rates.

Fires are more likely to occur in domestic than in non-domestic premises; this may be explained by the fire regulations that cover non-domestic premises such as factories or offices. There are about 45,000 fires in domestic dwellings in the UK each year.

There are a number of causes of fires in domestic dwellings, including, of course, arson. Open fires, cigarettes and candles are common triggers, as well as faulty electrical appliances and cooking equipment. People may not be able to escape from a fire if fire escapes are blocked or inadequate or if, for example, double-glazed windows are locked and the keys are not readily accessible.

Older people who live on their own, people with disabilities and people under the influence of alcohol are most vulnerable if a fire breaks out in their home. Babies and toddlers are also vulnerable as they are less able to escape from burning houses without assistance.

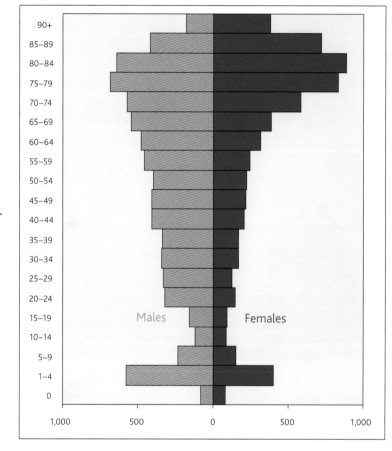

Fires in domestic homes can be prevented by enforcing housing standards, home safety checks and modifications, functioning alarms and advice and information to vulnerable groups.

Thirty-one people died in a fire at the King's Cross underground station in 1987.

ICD-9 codes: E890-E899
ICD-10 codes: X00-X06, X08-X09

ICD-9	ICD-9 name	% of cases	ICD-10	ICD-10 name	% of cases
E890	Conflagration in private dwelling	53.9	X00	Exposure to uncontrolled fire in building or structure	72.2
E893	Accident caused by ignition of clothing	7.8	X04	Exposure to ignition of highly flammable material	5.7
E898	Accident caused by other specified fire and flames	17.1			
E899	Accident caused by unspecified fire	9.9	X09	Exposure to unspecified smoke, fire and flames	8.7
	Other causes in group	11.3		Other causes in group	13.4
		100.0			100.0

MAP 43   FIRE

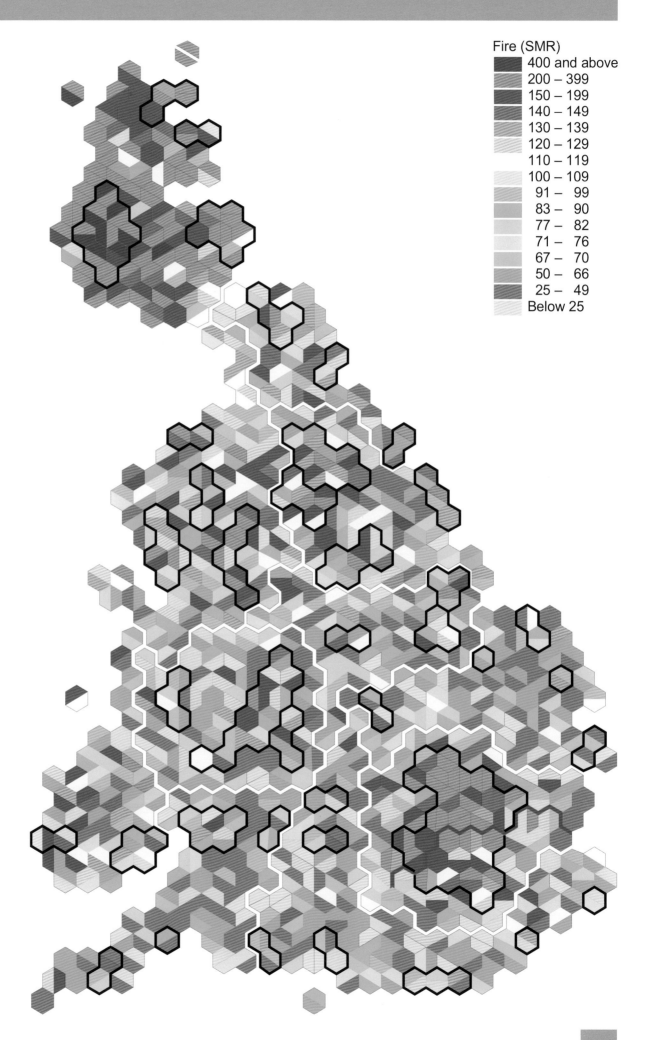

Fire (SMR)

- 400 and above
- 200 – 399
- 150 – 199
- 140 – 149
- 130 – 139
- 120 – 129
- 110 – 119
- 100 – 109
- 91 – 99
- 83 – 90
- 77 – 82
- 71 – 76
- 67 – 70
- 50 – 66
- 25 – 49
- Below 25

44 HEPATITIS

Hepatitis is inflammation of the cells of the liver. It can be acute, lasting for less than six months, or chronic when it lasts for longer. At its most severe hepatitis can lead to liver failure.

See Map 47 Chronic liver disease.

3,085 cases

0.02% of all deaths

average age = 56.0

male:female ratio = 67:33

Males and females are mapped separately as the geographical patterns are very different. Two thirds of deaths from hepatitis were of males. Both males and females have high SMRs in London, where nearly a quarter of all deaths from this cause occurred.

Hepatitis can be viral or non-viral. The most common forms of viral hepatitis are A, B and C.

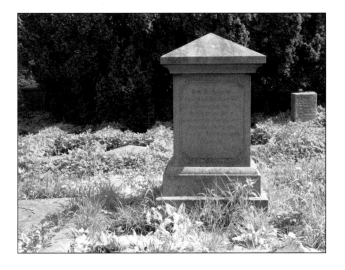

Hepatitis A, or infectious jaundice, causes an acute form of hepatitis. It is a virus transmitted by the faecal-oral route and is often associated with ingesting contaminated food. This is the commonest form of hepatitis, but is rarely fatal, and does not cause chronic liver disease. Most infections occur in childhood and pass unnoticed.

Hepatitis B can cause both acute and chronic hepatitis. Transmission can be via blood, by needles (used for tattoos or drugs), sexual or through breast-feeding. Hepatitis B is considered an occupational hazard for healthcare workers and the emergency services.

Hepatitis C can be transmitted through blood and can cross the placenta. It can remain asymptomatic for up to 20 years and culminate in cirrhosis. There is currently no vaccine for Hepatitis C.

Hepatitis B and C are a major health threat to injecting drug users.

In the late 1970s and early 1980s in Britain some 4,800 haemophiliacs were infected with Hepatitis C due to infected blood product transfusions (see www.taintedblood.info).

ICD-9 codes: 070
ICD-10 codes: B15-B19

ICD-9	ICD-9 name	% of cases	ICD-10	ICD-10 name	% of cases
070.1	Viral hepatitis A without mention of hepatic coma	8.7			
070.3	Viral hepatitis B without mention of hepatic coma	43.8	B16	Acute hepatitis B	20.6
070.5	Other specified viral hepatitis without mention of hepatic coma	23.0	B17	Other acute viral hepatitis	54.1
070.9	Unspecified viral hepatitis without mention of hepatic coma	20.6	B18	Chronic viral hepatitis	20.2
	Other causes in group	3.9		Other causes in group	5.1
		100.0			100.0

MAP 44A (FEMALES) 44B (MALES)　　HEPATITIS

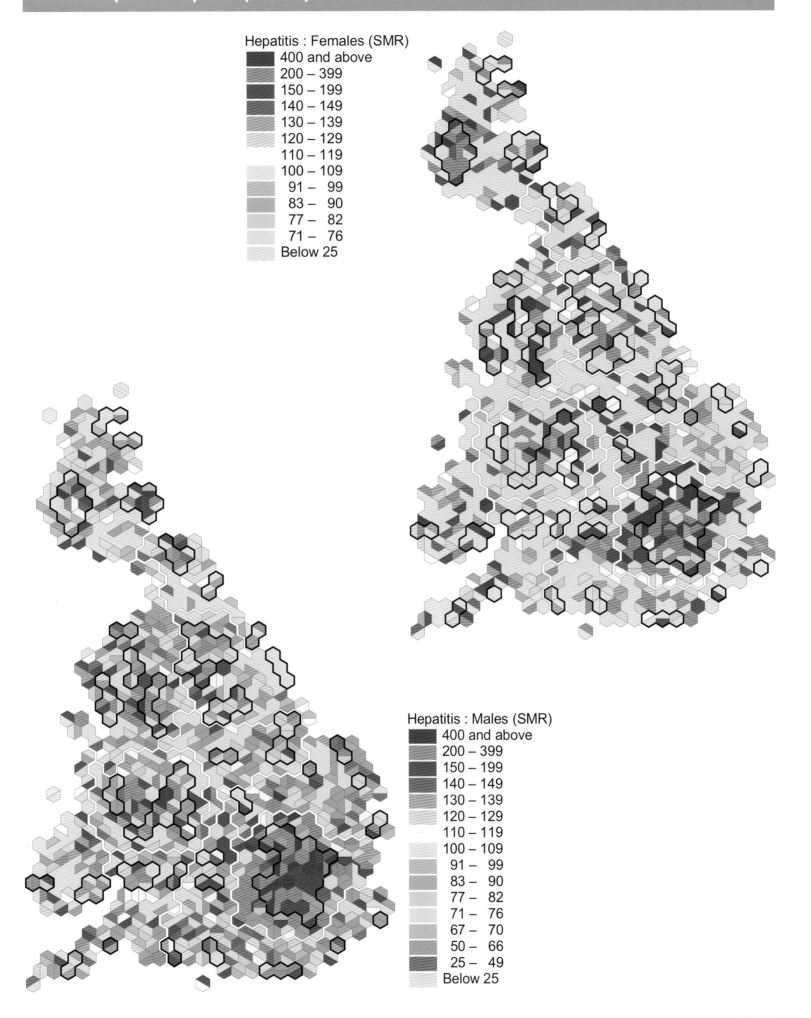

Hepatitis : Females (SMR)

- 400 and above
- 200 – 399
- 150 – 199
- 140 – 149
- 130 – 139
- 120 – 129
- 110 – 119
- 100 – 109
- 91 – 99
- 83 – 90
- 77 – 82
- 71 – 76
- Below 25

Hepatitis : Males (SMR)

- 400 and above
- 200 – 399
- 150 – 199
- 140 – 149
- 130 – 139
- 120 – 129
- 110 – 119
- 100 – 109
- 91 – 99
- 83 – 90
- 77 – 82
- 71 – 76
- 67 – 70
- 50 – 66
- 25 – 49
- Below 25

45 CHOKING ON FOOD

These deaths are those caused by choking on food or vomit.

See also Map 34 Suicide/undetermined by hanging, which includes deaths due to asphyxiation.

9,208 cases

0.06% of all deaths

average age = 57.4

male:female ratio = 53:47

Central and western Scotland are immediately obvious as the places with the highest SMRs. Outside of Scotland, Morpeth and St Albans East are the only neighbourhoods with SMRs over 400.

Choking is involuntary coughing or gasping for air caused by the blockage of the windpipe (trachea) which can occur when food goes down the windpipe rather than the food pipe (oesophagus). It is more unusual to choke on non-food objects.

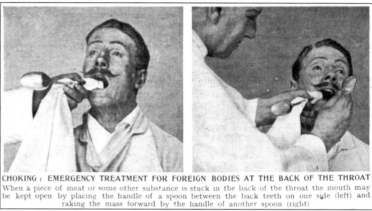

CHOKING : EMERGENCY TREATMENT FOR FOREIGN BODIES AT THE BACK OF THE THROAT
When a piece of meat or some other substance is stuck in the back of the throat the mouth may be kept open by placing the handle of a spoon between the back teeth on one side (left) and raking the mass forward by the handle of another spoon (right)

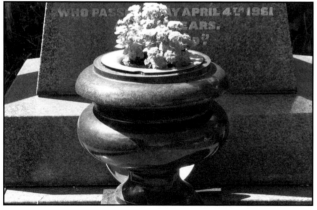

Choking can also be caused by the blockage of the airways by vomit. This form of choking is most often associated with excessive alcohol consumption. Rates are high in particular parts of some university towns where students are concentrated.

Musician Jimi Hendrix died from this cause.

It is well known that babies and toddlers are at a higher risk from this cause, but it can cause death to adults of all ages. Two-fifths of these deaths are of the over 70s. Fishbones, nuts, raisins, sweets, raw vegetables, burgers and steak are some of the most common foods involved in choking incidents; pretzels are less common although apparently almost claimed George W. Bush in 2002.

ICD-9 codes: E911
ICD-10 codes: W78-W79

ICD-9	ICD-9 name	% of cases	ICD-10	ICD-10 name	% of cases
E911	Inhalation and ingestion of food causing obstruction of respiratory tract or suffocation	100.0	W78	Inhalation of gastric contents	43.9
			W79	Inhalation and ingestion of food causing obstruction of respiratory tract	56.1
		100.0			100.0

MAP 45   CHOKING ON FOOD

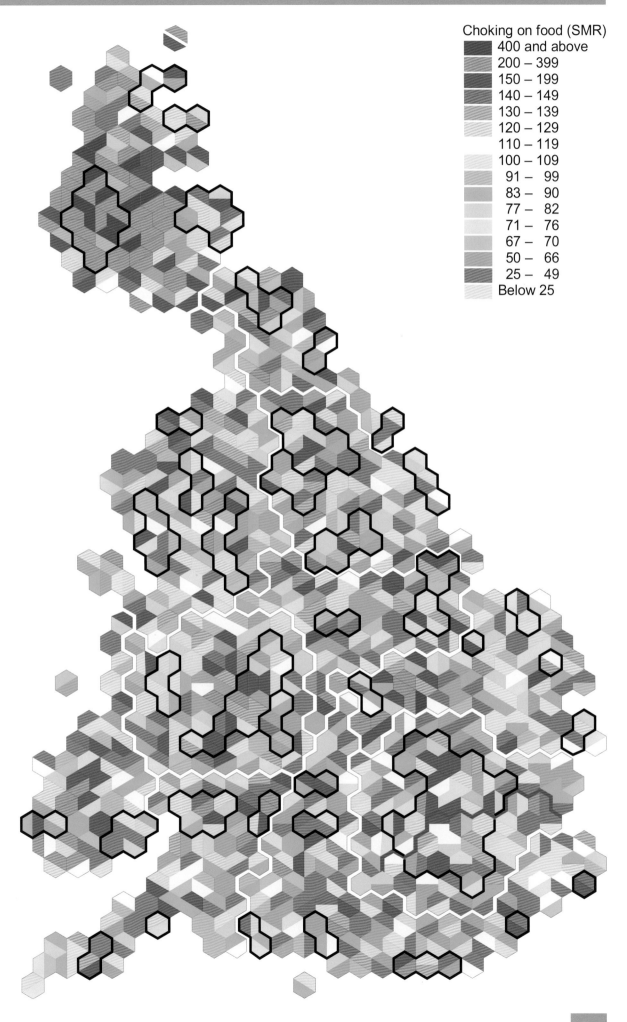

Choking on food (SMR)
- 400 and above
- 200 – 399
- 150 – 199
- 140 – 149
- 130 – 139
- 120 – 129
- 110 – 119
- 100 – 109
- 91 – 99
- 83 – 90
- 77 – 82
- 71 – 76
- 67 – 70
- 50 – 66
- 25 – 49
- Below 25

46 CANCER OF BRAIN

This is a sub-category of All cancer deaths (see Map 7). It refers to cancers that start within the brain, and does not include deaths from cancers that start elsewhere and spread to the brain.

68,431 cases

0.46% of all deaths

average age = 58.6

male:female ratio = 57:43

There appears to be little geographical patterning to deaths from brain cancer. Higher SMRs are found in a few areas – Glasgow and the north of Edinburgh – with slightly lower rates in the south of Aberdeen and around Berwickshire. Within England and Wales there is a slight north–south divide with the southern part seeing slightly higher rates. Rates also tend to be slightly lower in the poorer parts of many cities and are slightly higher than average in those parts of the Home Counties nearest to London.

Brain tumours account for less than 2% of primary tumours in cancer, but 7% of years of life lost from cancer before age 70 (Cancer Research UK).

The commonest symptoms of brain tumours are headaches and fits (although brain tumours are a rare cause of headaches and fits: there is usually an alternative explanation for these symptoms).

There are nearly 100 different types of brain tumour. They tend to be named after the type of cell they developed from or the area of the brain in which they are located. It is not known what causes most brain tumours; the only known causal factor is exposure to radioactivity.

Politicians Mo Mowlam and Alan Clark and actor Brian Glover died from this cause.

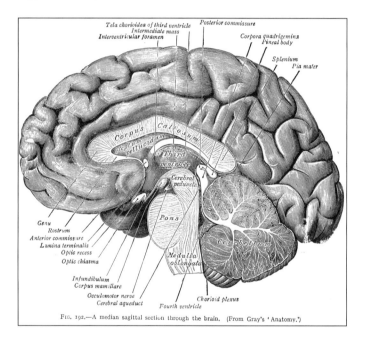

FIG. 192.—A median sagittal section through the brain. (From Gray's 'Anatomy.')

ICD-9 codes: 191
ICD-10 codes: C71

ICD-9	ICD-9 name	% of cases	ICD-10	ICD-10 name	% of cases
191	Malignant neoplasm of brain	100.0	C71	Malignant neoplasm of brain	100.0
		100.0			100.0

MAP 46   CANCER OF BRAIN

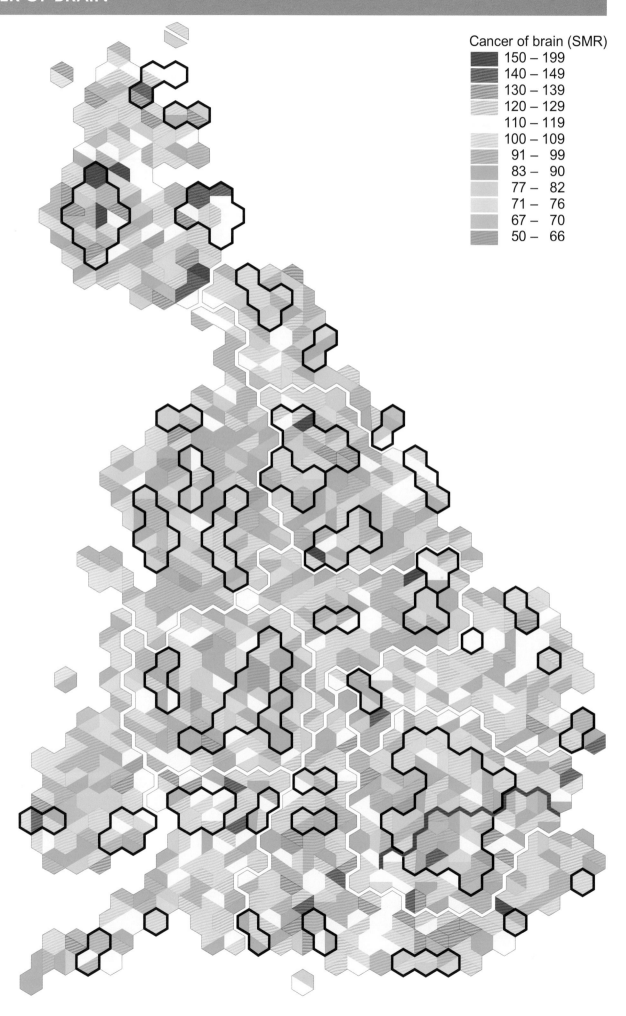

Cancer of brain (SMR)
- 150 – 199
- 140 – 149
- 130 – 139
- 120 – 129
- 110 – 119
- 100 – 109
- 91 – 99
- 83 – 90
- 77 – 82
- 71 – 76
- 67 – 70
- 50 – 66

47 CHRONIC LIVER DISEASE

Chronic liver disease is the gradual destruction of the liver over time. It is a cause of death that includes cirrhosis and fibrosis of the liver and also alcoholic liver disease – which accounts for two thirds of the deaths due to this cause.

See also Map 40 Due to alcohol, and Map 44 Hepatitis.

100,933 cases

0.68% of all deaths

average age = 59.0

male:female ratio = 59:41

Scotland, particularly Glasgow, sees the highest rates, with male rates higher than female. Inner London and the north west of England also see high rates for both sexes. In addition, there are also male clusters in Newcastle and south Wales. Rates are dramatically low in East Anglia and much of southern England. In general there is a very clear geographical divide.

Chronic liver disease can lead to cirrhosis of the liver, which is the replacement of normal liver tissue by fibrous scar tissue and regenerative nodules leading to progressive loss of liver function. Fibrosis is the formation of excess fibrous connective tissues.

Alcohol consumption and hepatitis are the most common causes of chronic liver disease. Together with the central nervous system, the liver is the part of the body most affected by alcohol consumption.

Forty-three per cent of deaths from this cause are of men aged 40–69.

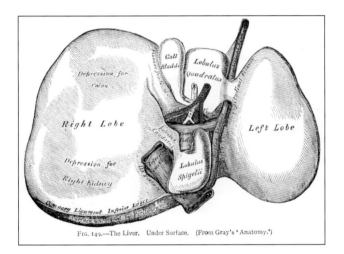

FIG. 140.—The Liver. Under Surface. (From Gray's 'Anatomy.')

ICD-9 codes: 571
ICD-10 codes: K70, K73-K74, K76.0

ICD-9	ICD-9 name	% of cases	ICD-10	ICD-10 name	% of cases
571	Chronic liver disease and cirrhosis	100.0	K70	Alcoholic liver disease	68.0
			K74	Fibrosis and cirrhosis of liver	26.9
				Other causes in group	5.1
		100.0			100.0

MAP 47A (FEMALES) 47B (MALES)   CHRONIC LIVER DISEASE

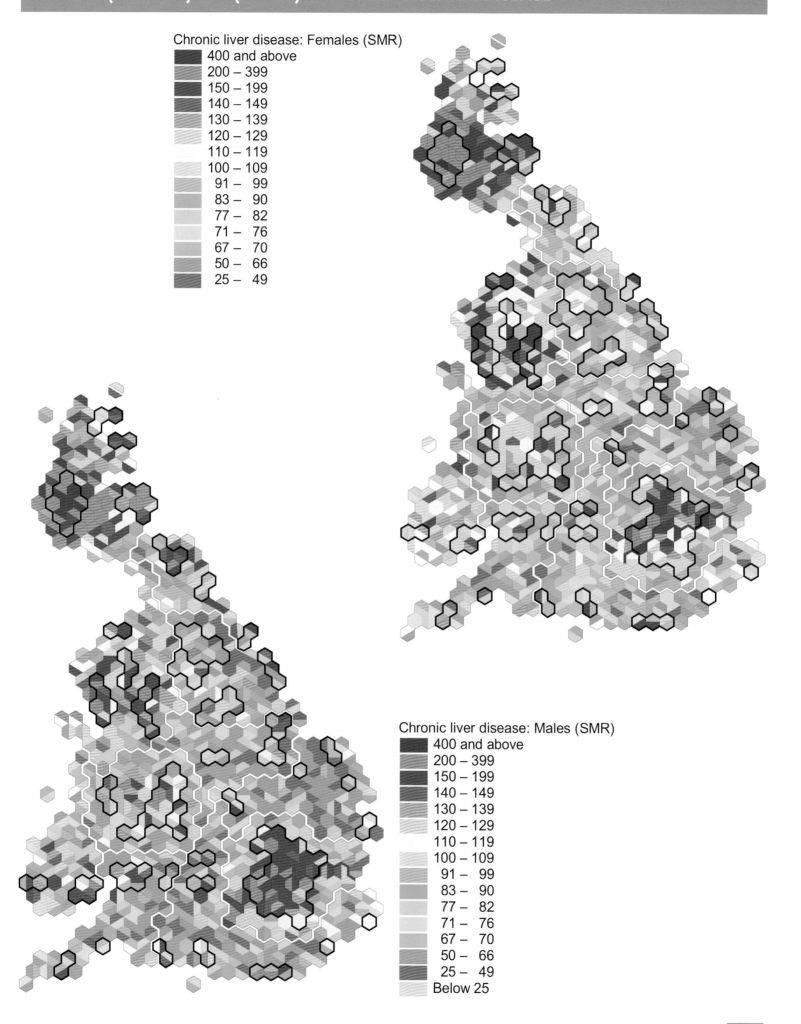

Chronic liver disease: Females (SMR)

- 400 and above
- 200 – 399
- 150 – 199
- 140 – 149
- 130 – 139
- 120 – 129
- 110 – 119
- 100 – 109
- 91 – 99
- 83 – 90
- 77 – 82
- 71 – 76
- 67 – 70
- 50 – 66
- 25 – 49

Chronic liver disease: Males (SMR)

- 400 and above
- 200 – 399
- 150 – 199
- 140 – 149
- 130 – 139
- 120 – 129
- 110 – 119
- 100 – 109
- 91 – 99
- 83 – 90
- 77 – 82
- 71 – 76
- 67 – 70
- 50 – 66
- 25 – 49
- Below 25

48 MULTIPLE SCLEROSIS

Multiple sclerosis, or MS, is a chronic disease of the central nervous system.

See also Map 56 Motor neurone disease.

> 21,275 cases
>
> 0.14% of all deaths
>
> average age = 59.4
>
> male:female ratio = 36:64

The highest rate of mortality attributed to MS is found in Putney West. The Royal Hospital for Neurodisability is found here: the high rate may be due to deaths of residents of that hospital. There are other clusters in the northernmost parts of Scotland and in the Scottish borders. This condition is twice as likely to occur among women than men. It is most often diagnosed between the ages of 20 and 40 (see age–sex bar chart).

MS results from damage to myelin – the protective sheath surrounding the nerve fibres within the central nervous system. This damage interferes with the communication of messages between the brain and parts of the body.

There are a variety of symptoms of MS, including changes in sensation, muscle weakness, abnormal muscle spasms, difficulty moving, coordination and balance, problems with speech or swallowing, visual problems, fatigue, acute or chronic pain syndromes, bladder and bowel difficulties, cognitive impairment and clinical depression.

Life with MS can vary greatly between individuals. Some people have periods of relapse and remission whereas for others the pathway is more progressive. MS is best seen as a lifelong condition rather than as a terminal illness.

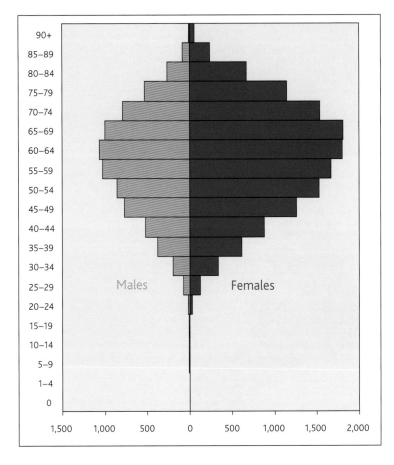

Cellist Jacqueline du Pre died from MS in 1987, aged 42.

ICD-9 codes: 340
ICD-10 codes: G35

ICD-9	ICD-9 name	% of cases	ICD-10	ICD-10 name	% of cases
340	Multiple sclerosis	100.0	G35	Multiple sclerosis	100.0
		100.0			100.0

MAP 48   MULTIPLE SCLEROSIS

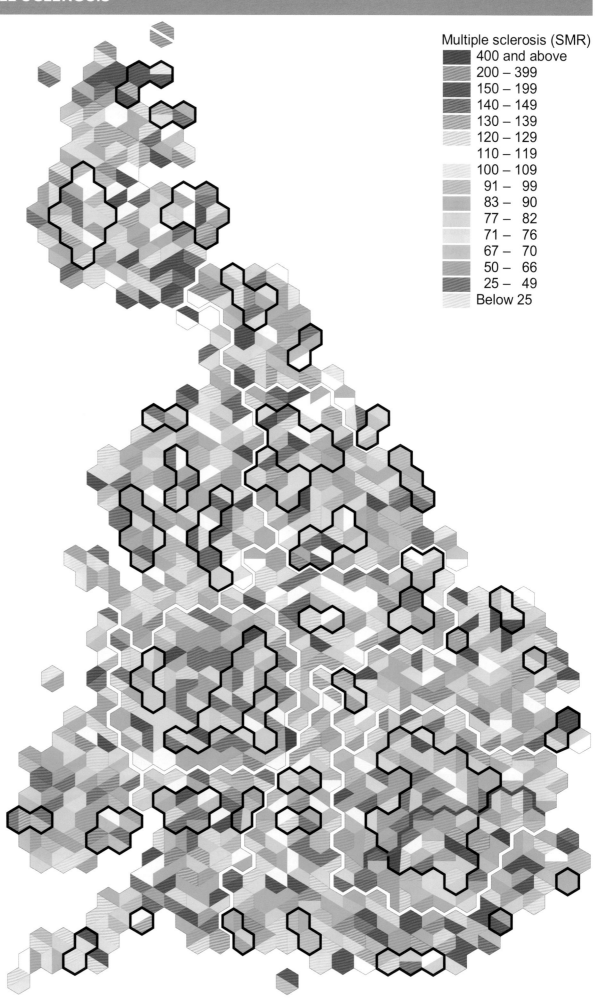

Multiple sclerosis (SMR)
- 400 and above
- 200 – 399
- 150 – 199
- 140 – 149
- 130 – 139
- 120 – 129
- 110 – 119
- 100 – 109
- 91 – 99
- 83 – 90
- 77 – 82
- 71 – 76
- 67 – 70
- 50 – 66
- 25 – 49
- Below 25

51   ILL-DEFINED AND UNKNOWN CAUSES

This cause of death is used when the cause of mortality in the deceased is not known and when there is no other cause that is deemed appropriate.

See also Map 80 Signs and symptoms.

11,698 cases

0.08% of all deaths

average age = 62.0

male:female ratio = 54:46

For males, the highest rates are clustered in central London, with a further cluster in the extreme north west of Scotland. For females, the highest rates are in the north west of Scotland, followed by North Ayrshire and the Tweeddale area. Forty per cent of deaths were of people aged over 75; females dominate these older age groups.

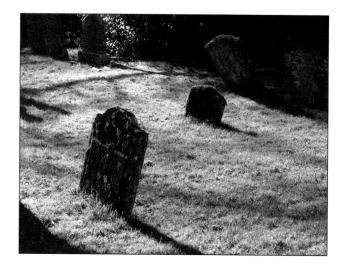

Despite advances in pathology, it is not always possible to determine the cause of a person's death. Some of these deaths will be the result of a corpse not being found for some time after death, meaning that there is insufficient evidence for the cause of death to be ascertained.

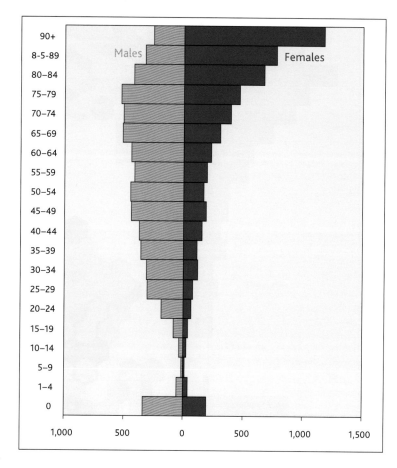

ICD-9 codes: 799
ICD-10 codes: R09.0, R09.2, R29, R64

ICD-9	ICD-9 name	% of cases	ICD-10	ICD-10 name	% of cases
799	Other ill-defined and unknown causes of morbidity and mortality	100.0	R09.2	Respiratory arrest	80.8
			R64	Cachexia	12.8
				Other causes in group	6.4
		100.0			100.0

MAP 51A (FEMALES) 51B (MALES)   ILL-DEFINED AND UNKNOWN CAUSES

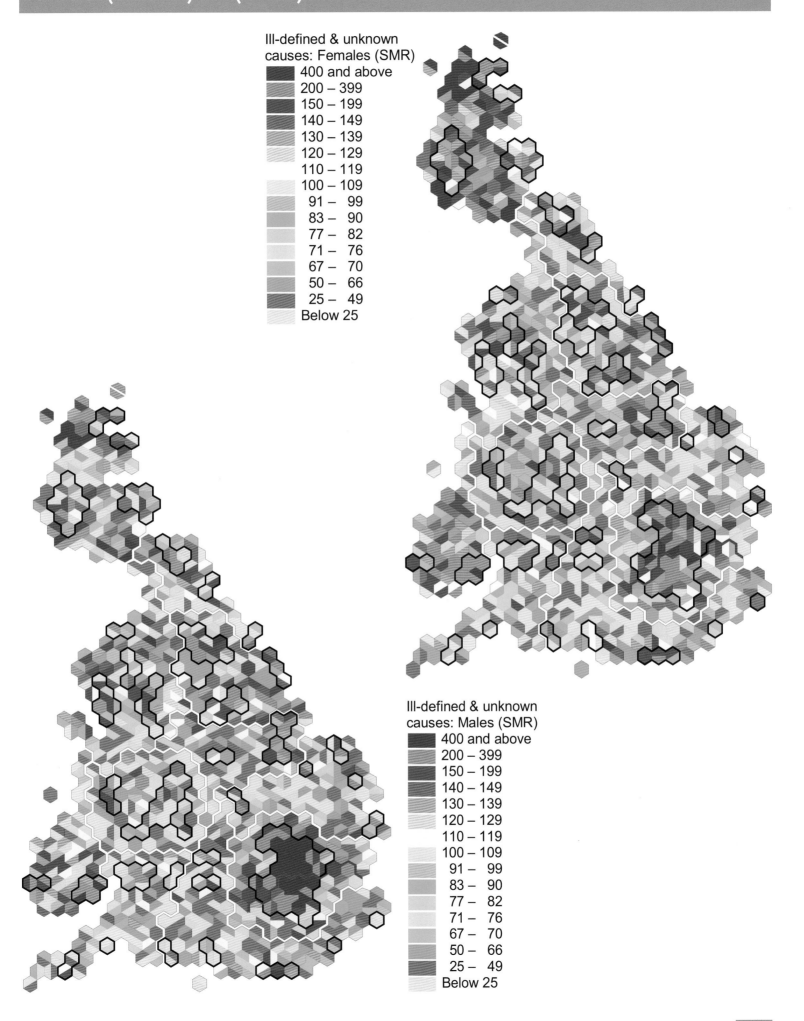

Ill-defined & unknown
causes: Females (SMR)

- 400 and above
- 200 – 399
- 150 – 199
- 140 – 149
- 130 – 139
- 120 – 129
- 110 – 119
- 100 – 109
- 91 – 99
- 83 – 90
- 77 – 82
- 71 – 76
- 67 – 70
- 50 – 66
- 25 – 49
- Below 25

Ill-defined & unknown
causes: Males (SMR)

- 400 and above
- 200 – 399
- 150 – 199
- 140 – 149
- 130 – 139
- 120 – 129
- 110 – 119
- 100 – 109
- 91 – 99
- 83 – 90
- 77 – 82
- 71 – 76
- 67 – 70
- 50 – 66
- 25 – 49
- Below 25

52   OTHER EXTERNAL CAUSES

This is a residual category and includes all external causes of death not included in categories elsewhere.

See also Map 5 All external deaths.

38,566 cases

0.26% of all deaths

average age = 62.0

male:female ratio = 55:45

On both the male and female maps, south and mid Wales are immediately striking. The highest SMRs for females are clustered around Mansfield, followed by Lancashire, Nottingham and the Jurassic coast area of southern England. Male clusters are found in London, Cambridge, Northampton and Bedford.

This category includes a veritable assortment of miscellaneous accidental causes of death, such as: complications associated with artificial fertilisation; collisions involving animals, riders of animals, or horse-drawn vehicles; falls involving ice-skates, skis, roller-skates or skateboards; being struck by a falling object or sports equipment; contact with a non-powered hand tool (for example, axe, can-opener, chisel); contact with a powered lawnmower; contact with powered hand tools and household machinery (for example, chainsaw, sewing machine); explosion and rupture of pressurised tyre, pipe or hose; foreign body entering into or through eye or other natural orifice; foreign body or object entering through skin; striking against or bumping into another person; being bitten or struck by dog or other mammal; being bitten or stung by non-venomous insect or other non-venomous arthropods; contact with plant thorns, spines or sharp leaves; accidental suffocation and strangulation in bed; being confined to or trapped in a low-oxygen environment; exposure to excessive heat, cold or high or low air pressure; contact with hot drinks, hot water or other hot fluids; contact with hot household appliances, radiators or pipes; contact with hornets, wasps and bees; contact with venomous arthropods; exposure to excessive natural heat (includes sunstroke); victim of lightning, avalanche, landslide or other earth movements; and overexertion and strenuous or repetitive movements (such as marathon running, rowing).

Excluding unspecified cause, the largest single cause of death in this category is death due to accidental suffocation (including accidental strangulation), accounting for 11% of deaths.

ICD-9 codes: E826.2, E826.6-E826.7, E826.9, E827-E829, E846, E848, E900, E902-E903, E905-E909, E912-E913, E915-E918, E920-E924, E927-E939, E941-E949, E970, E974-E977, E994, E997-E999

ICD-10 codes: N98, V09.9, V80.0, V80.7-V80.9, V82-V83, W02, W20-W23, W25-W29, W33-W34, W37, W39-W40, W44-W45, W49-W51, W54-W55, W57, W60, W64, W75-W77, W80-W81, W83-W84, W92, W94, X10-X12, X15-X16, X19, X23, X25, X30, X32-X33, X36, X39, X50, X58-X59, Y35, Y40-Y45, Y47-Y49, Y52-Y57, Y85-Y86, Y89

ICD-9	ICD-9 name	% of cases	ICD-10	ICD-10 name	% of cases
E913	Accidental mechanical suffocation	11.3			
E916	Struck accidentally by falling object	5.4			
E928	Other and unspecified environmental and accidental causes	53.6	X59	Exposure to unspecified factor	83.9
E929	Late effects of accidental injury	7.1			
	Other causes in group	22.6		Other causes in group	16.1
		100.0			100.0

MAP 52A (FEMALES) 52B (MALES) OTHER EXTERNAL CAUSES

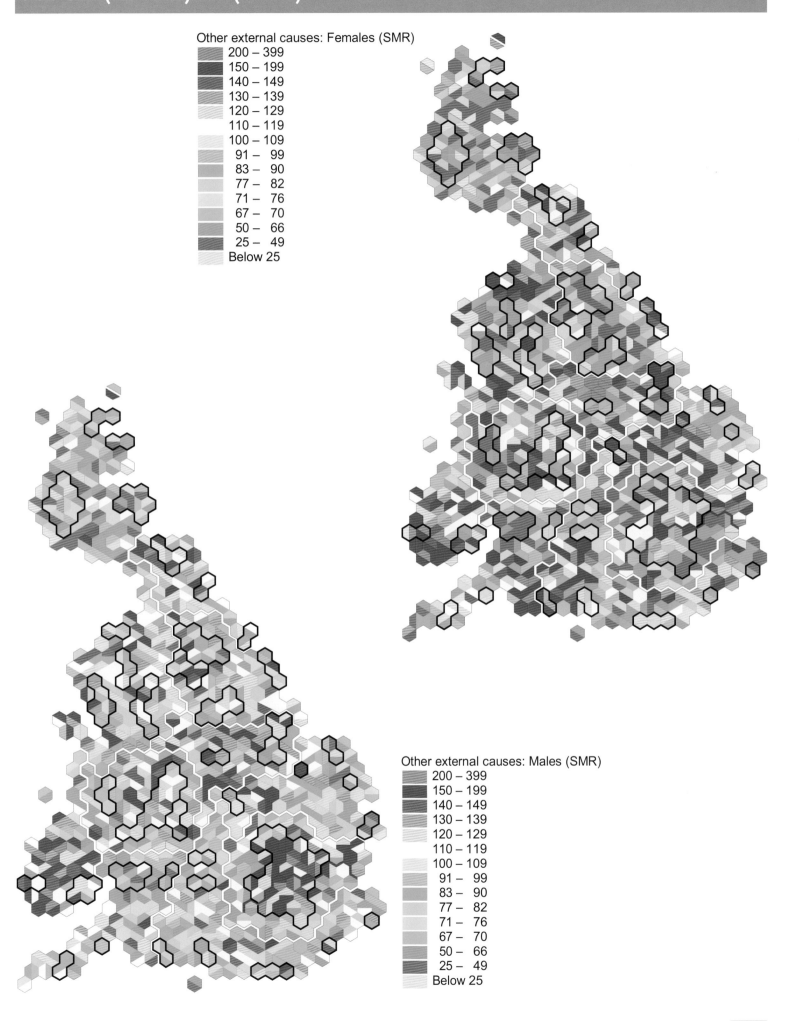

Other external causes: Females (SMR)
- 200 – 399
- 150 – 199
- 140 – 149
- 130 – 139
- 120 – 129
- 110 – 119
- 100 – 109
- 91 – 99
- 83 – 90
- 77 – 82
- 71 – 76
- 67 – 70
- 50 – 66
- 25 – 49
- Below 25

Other external causes: Males (SMR)
- 200 – 399
- 150 – 199
- 140 – 149
- 130 – 139
- 120 – 129
- 110 – 119
- 100 – 109
- 91 – 99
- 83 – 90
- 77 – 82
- 71 – 76
- 67 – 70
- 50 – 66
- 25 – 49
- Below 25

53 CERVICAL CANCER

This is a sub-category of cancer (see Map 7 All cancer deaths).

See also Map 59 Ovarian cancer, Map 62 Breast cancer and Map 76 Other uterine cancer.

40,094 cases

0.27% of all deaths

average age = 62.0

male:female ratio = 0:100

The prominent cluster of high SMRs is seen in a belt stretching across the north of England from Merseyside in the west across to Grimsby in the east. There are high rates in parts of Scotland and south Wales. Rates are very low, apart from in central London, south of a line extending from the Bristol Channel to the Wash.

Cervical cancer, or cancer of the cervix, affects the lower, narrow portion of the uterus. The early stage of this cancer is usually asymptomatic but it is detectable by examining cells removed from the cervix via a cervical smear, also known as a pap smear.

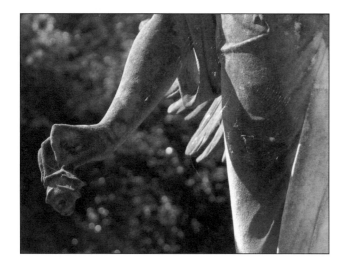

Women who have been exposed to some sexually transmitted strains of the human papillomavirus (HPV) are at increased risk of cervical cancer. These strains are responsible for the large majority of cervical cancers. Human papillomaviruses cause warts but infection may occur without warts being noticed. Other risk factors include smoking, HIV infection, chlamydia infection, dietary factors, hormonal contraception, multiple pregnancies and a family history of cervical cancer.

The NHS introduced a national screening programme for cervical cancer in 1988. Under this programme all women aged between 25 and 64 are eligible for a free cervical screening test every three to five years. Routine HPV vaccination was introduced in the UK from September 2008 for girls aged 12–13 as part of a national immunisation programme.

Over the 24 years covered by this atlas, the number of women dying from cervical cancer has halved.

First Lady of Argentina Eva Peron died from this cause.

ICD-9 codes: 180
ICD-10 codes: C53

ICD-9	ICD-9 name	% of cases	ICD-10	ICD-10 name	% of cases
180	Malignant neoplasm of cervix uteri	100.0	C53	Malignant neoplasm of cervix uteri	100.0
		100.0			100.0

MAP 53   CERVICAL CANCER

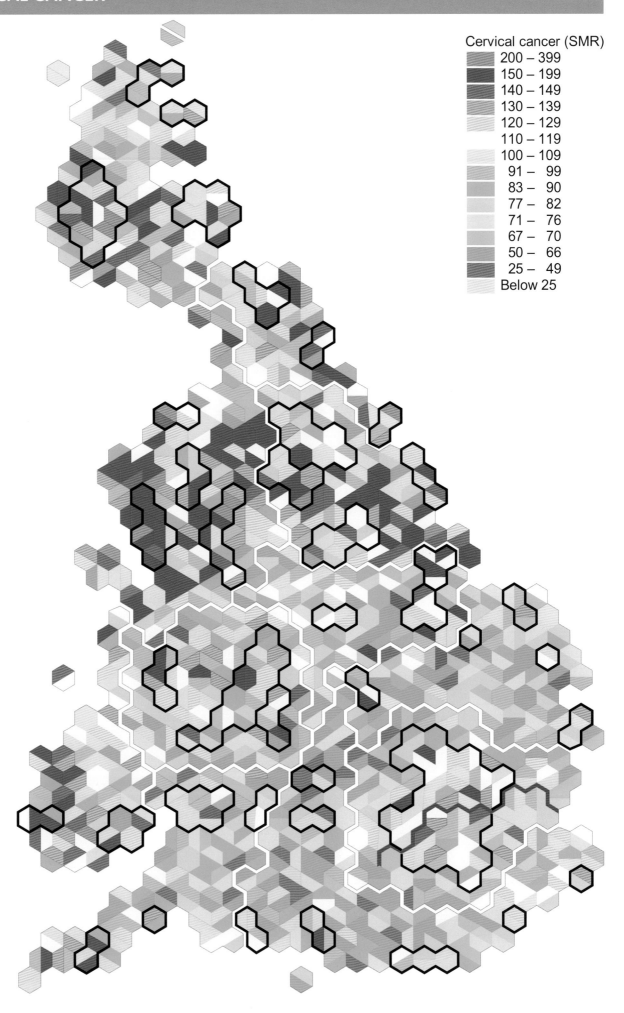

Cervical cancer (SMR)
- 200 – 399
- 150 – 199
- 140 – 149
- 130 – 139
- 120 – 129
- 110 – 119
- 100 – 109
- 91 – 99
- 83 – 90
- 77 – 82
- 71 – 76
- 67 – 70
- 50 – 66
- 25 – 49
- Below 25

54 SKIN CANCER

This is a sub-category of all cancer deaths (see Map 7) and includes only the form of skin cancer known as malignant melanoma.

See also Other neoplasms (Map 61), which includes other forms of skin cancer.

32,884 cases

0.22% of all deaths

average age = 63.4

male:female ratio = 49:51

There is an obvious north-south divide on the map, with a gradient from higher rates on the south coast to lower rates in northern parts. This probably reflects the British climate, and also where those who can afford to holiday in the sun reside.

Malignant melanoma, the form of skin cancer that we map here, is the most serious type of skin cancer as it can spread to other parts of the body. The leading cause of skin cancer is over-exposure to sunlight. Rates have been increasing in recent years, thought to be due to increasing numbers of people taking increasing numbers of holidays abroad, and the popularity of the 'tanned look' and the use of tanning booths and sun lamps to achieve that look.

Skin cancer is very evenly distributed between males and females (see age–sex bar chart) although the age distributions are slightly different. For both males and females mortality increases incrementally with age until the 70s, reflecting, possibly, accumulated sun exposure over the life course.

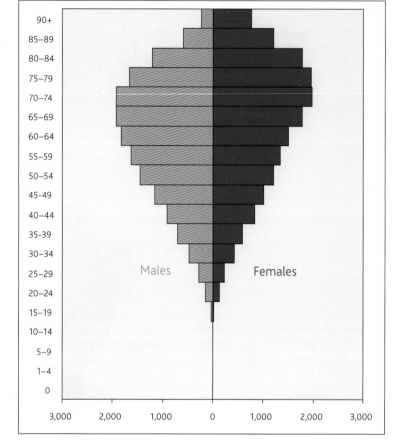

ICD-9 codes: 172
ICD-10 codes: C43

ICD-9	ICD-9 name	% of cases	ICD-10	ICD-10 name	% of cases
172	Malignant melanoma of skin	100.0	C43	Malignant melanoma of skin	100.0
		100.0			100.0

MAP 54   SKIN CANCER

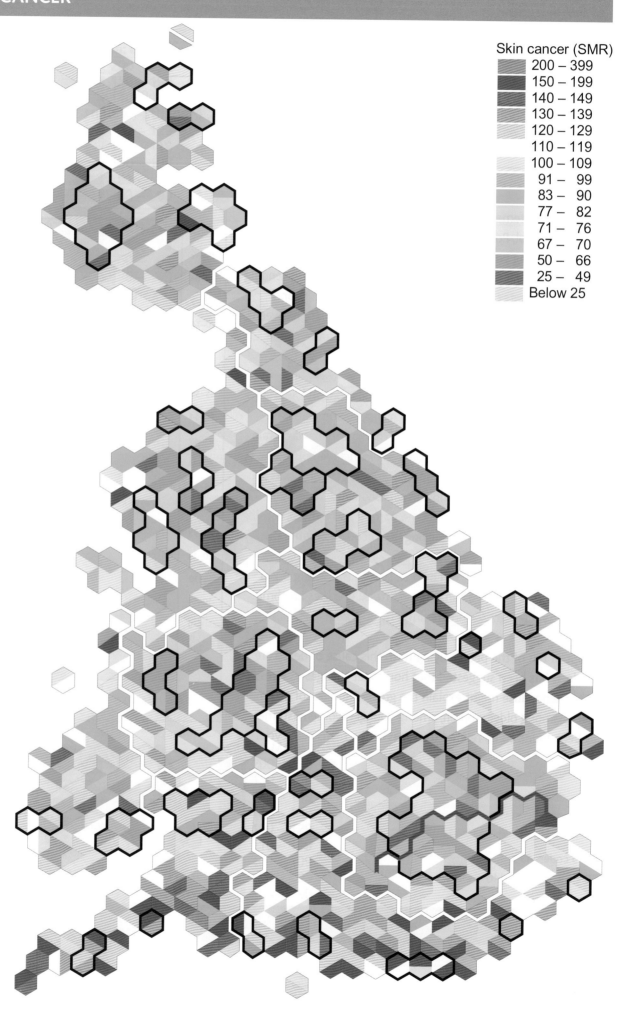

Skin cancer (SMR)
- 200 – 399
- 150 – 199
- 140 – 149
- 130 – 139
- 120 – 129
- 110 – 119
- 100 – 109
- 91 – 99
- 83 – 90
- 77 – 82
- 71 – 76
- 67 – 70
- 50 – 66
- 25 – 49
- Below 25

57 ENDOCRINE DISORDERS (NOT DIABETES)

The diseases in this category are the result of disorders of the endocrine system. This system releases hormones into the blood from the endocrine glands and tissues. Hormones are molecules that send signals from one type of cell to another. There are hundreds of different types of endocrine disorders.

See also Map 85 Diabetes mellitus.

45,844 cases

0.31% of all deaths

average age = 66.5

male:female ratio = 38:62

Clusters of high SMRs are found in and around Birmingham and in the south Wales valleys. Scotland also has high rates. Low rates are found in more affluent areas where wealthier older people retire.

This cause of death is more common for females than for males, with 62% of all deaths from these causes being of females. As the age–sex bar chart shows, it is women over the age of 60 who are most likely to die from these causes.

Nearly a quarter of deaths in this grouping are due to thyroid problems. Just over a tenth (11.2% for ICD-10) of the deaths in this category are due to morbid obesity. Also included here is cystic fibrosis, which is a hereditary disease causing progressive disability affecting the lungs and digestive system. Morbid obesity is defined as a body mass index of more than 35kg/m^2. A BMI of between 25–35 carries increased mortality risk but would not be recorded as cause of death. When noted as a cause of death, the BMI is likely to be well over 35.

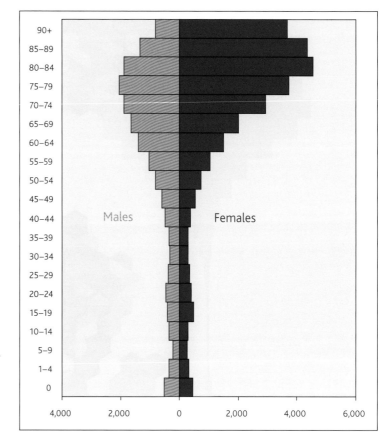

ICD-9 codes: 240-246, 251-278

ICD-10 codes: C88.0, C88.2, D44.8, D47.2, D76, D89.0-D89.1, E00, E03.1-E03.2, E03.4, E03.9, E04-E07, E15-E16, E20-E27, E31-E32, E34, E41, E43, E46, E51, E53, E55, E61, E63-E64, E66, E70-E72, E74, E75.2, E75.5-E75.6, E76-E80, E83-E88, M10, M83

ICD-9	ICD-9 name	% of cases	ICD-10	ICD-10 name	% of cases
242	Thyrotoxicosis with or without goitre	6.1			
244.9	Unspecified hypothyroidism	16.6	E03.9	Hypothyroidism, unspecified	13.2
272	Disorders of lipoid metabolism	5.9	E78	Disorders of lipoprotein metabolism and other lipidaemias	7.1
273	Disorders of plasma protein metabolism	7.3	C88.0	Waldenström's macroglobulinaemia	5.8
276	Disorders of fluid, electrolyte and acid-base balance	11.8	E86	Volume depletion	9.2
			E87	Other disorders of fluid, electrolyte and acid-base balance	5.9
277	Other and unspecified disorders of metabolism	18.1	E84	Cystic fibrosis	6.1
			E85	Amyloidosis	9.1
278	Obesity and other hyperalimentation	10.6	E66	Obesity	11.3
	Other causes in group	23.6		Other causes in group	32.3
		100.0			100.0

MAP 57   ENDOCRINE DISORDERS (NOT DIABETES)

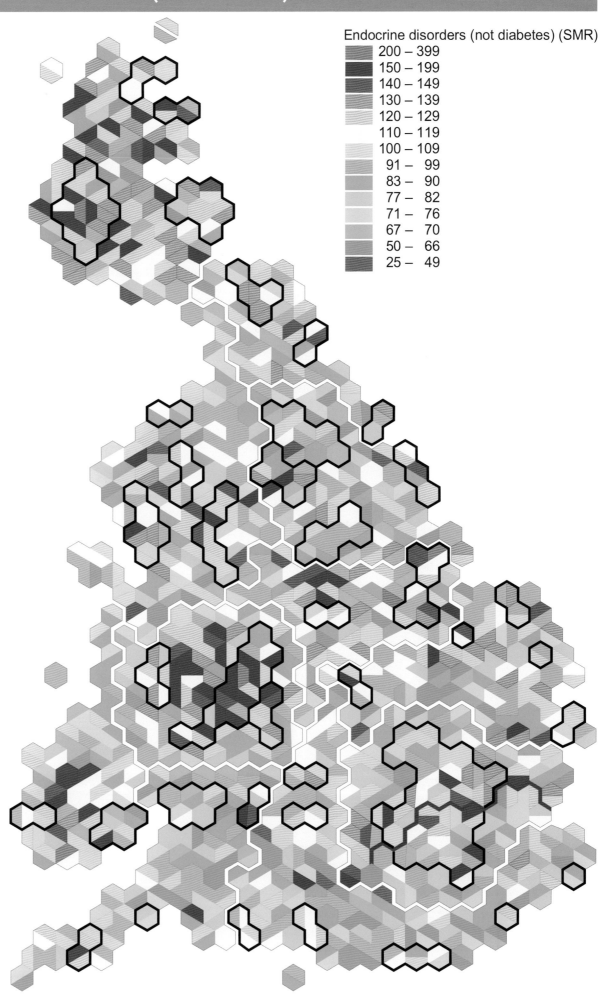

Endocrine disorders (not diabetes) (SMR)

- 200 – 399
- 150 – 199
- 140 – 149
- 130 – 139
- 120 – 129
- 110 – 119
- 100 – 109
- 91 – 99
- 83 – 90
- 77 – 82
- 71 – 76
- 67 – 70
- 50 – 66
- 25 – 49

58   LEUKAEMIA

Leukaemia is cancer of the blood or bone marrow. This is a broad range of diseases including both acute and chronic forms.

See also Map 7 All cancer deaths.

93,048 cases

0.63% of all deaths

average age = 67.2

male:female ratio = 54:46

SMRs are generally slightly lower north of a line running from the mouth of the Mersey to the Thames estuary. The highest SMRs are found in Wigan, Northampton, Newport Pagnell and Burnley. In general the distribution is much more even than for most other causes of death.

Childhood leukaemia is the most common form of childhood malignancy, with acute lymphoblastic leukaemia accounting for approximately three quarters of childhood leukaemias, with incidence peaking between ages 2 and 3. However, as the age–sex bar chart shows, it is older adults who are much more likely to die from this group of cancers than young people. In these older age groups the forms of the disease that are prevalent are chronic lymphocytic leukaemia and myeloid leukaemia.

Survival rates have improved dramatically in recent years. Approximately 75% of all children with childhood cancers survive five years after diagnosis, with the figure being 80% for those with acute lymphoblastic leukaemia (UK Childhood Cancer Research Group, National Registry of Childhood Tumours, 2004). Most of these will be permanently cured.

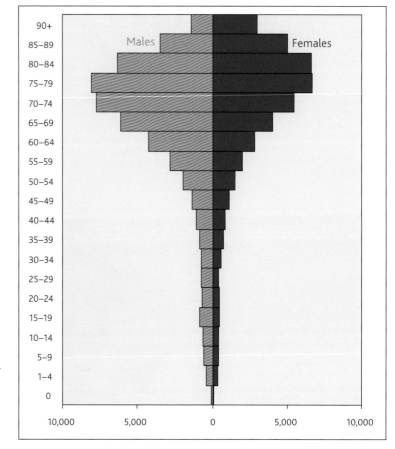

ICD-9 codes: 204-208
ICD-10 codes: C91.0-C91.1, C91.3, C91.5, C91.9, C92-C95

ICD-9	ICD-9 name	% of cases	ICD-10	ICD-10 name	% of cases
204	Lymphoid leukaemia - Acute	8.5	C91.0	Acute lymphoblastic leukaemia	7.0
204.1	Lymphoid leukaemia - Chronic	23.2	C91.1	Chronic lymphocytic leukaemia	24.5
205	Myeloid leukaemia	56.6	C92	Myeloid leukaemia	60.3
208	Leukaemia of unspecified cell type	7.9	C95	Leukaemia of unspecified cell type	6.0
	Other causes in group	3.8		Other causes in group	2.2
		100.0			100.0

MAP 58   LEUKAEMIA

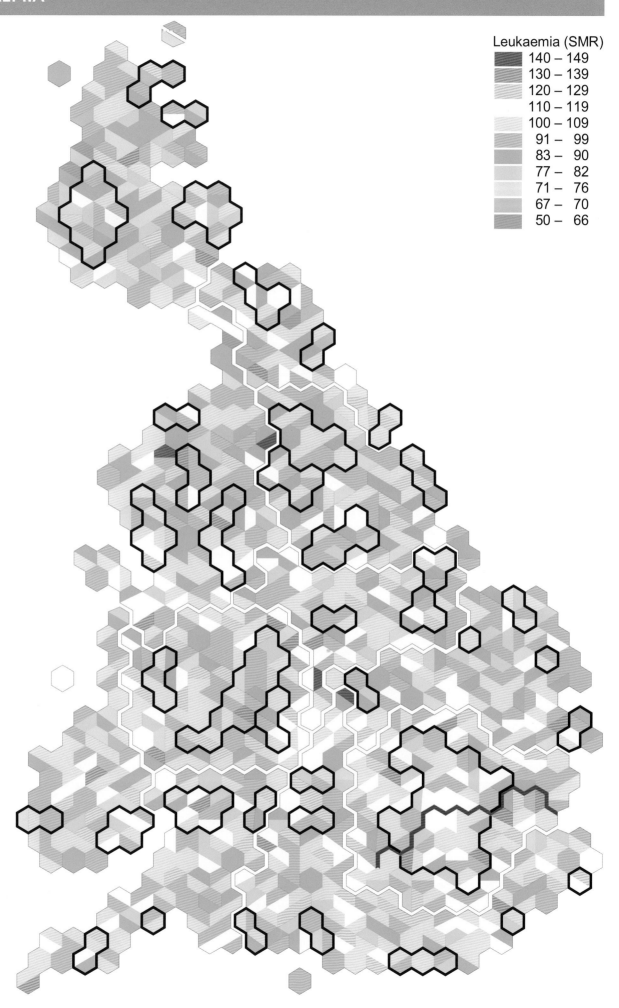

Leukaemia (SMR)
- 140 – 149
- 130 – 139
- 120 – 129
- 110 – 119
- 100 – 109
- 91 – 99
- 83 – 90
- 77 – 82
- 71 – 76
- 67 – 70
- 50 – 66

59   OVARIAN CANCER

This is a sub-category of cancer (see Map 7 All cancer deaths).

See also Map 53 Cervical cancer, Map 62 Breast cancer and Map 76 Other uterine cancer.

102,206 cases

0.68% of all deaths

average age = 67.6

male:female ratio = 0:100

There is little geographical patterning to mortality from ovarian cancer. The highest rates are found in the urban parts of Montgomeryshire, Ettrick and Lauderdale, North East Dorset and the rural parts of the Wrekin. Even for these areas, the SMR is only one and a half times the national average. However, there is clear, if slight, urban/suburban–rural differentiation in the West Midlands and around Greater London – with rates higher outside of the cities. This patterning coincides well with age of motherhood geographies; mothers tend on average to be older at the time of birth of their children in the south of England and the more affluent suburbs of cities.

Ovarian cancer is a malignant tumour of the ovary. The exact cause of ovarian cancer is unknown, but is strongly familial. The risk is increased by having many ovulations. A woman has fewer ovulations if her periods start later, if she has children and if she uses low-dose hormonal contraceptives.

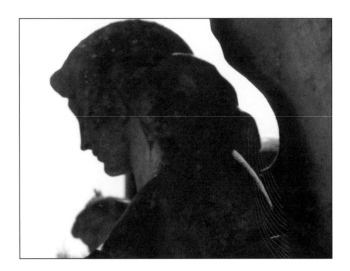

The comedian Linda Smith died of ovarian cancer.

ICD-9 codes: 183
ICD-10 codes: C56, C57.0-C57.1

ICD-9	ICD-9 name	% of cases	ICD-10	ICD-10 name	% of cases
183	Malignant neoplasm of ovary and other uterine adnexa	100.0	C56	Malignant neoplasm of ovary	99.4
				Other causes in group	0.6
		100.0			100.0

MAP 59   OVARIAN CANCER

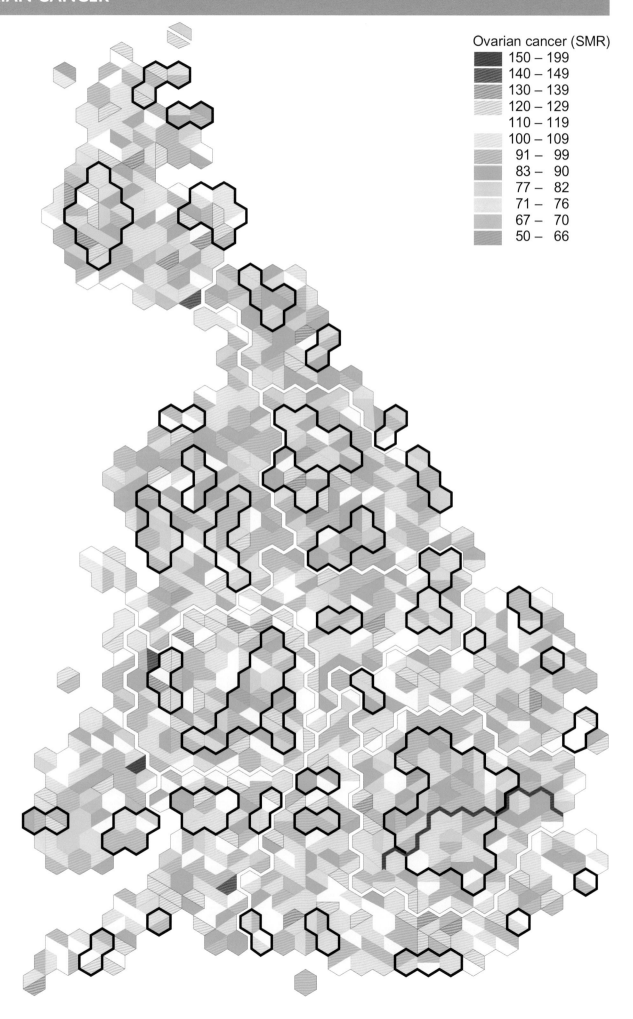

Ovarian cancer (SMR)

■	150 – 199
▨	140 – 149
▨	130 – 139
▨	120 – 129
	110 – 119
▨	100 – 109
▨	91 – 99
▨	83 – 90
▨	77 – 82
▨	71 – 76
▨	67 – 70
▨	50 – 66

60   CANCER OF THE MOUTH

Also known as oral cancer, this category includes any cancerous tissue growth located in the mouth.

See also Map 7 All cancer deaths, Map 65 Laryngeal cancer and Map 71 Cancer of gullet.

45,391 cases

0.31% of all deaths

average age = 67.7

male:female ratio = 63:37

Compare this map to Map 47B (chronic liver disease, males) and Map 68 (lung cancer). They have very similar patterns, and this map could almost be a map of the combined effects of smoking and drinking. The west of Scotland, Edinburgh, the urban parts of north west England, Newcastle-upon-Tyne, and London north of the Thames all have high rates. In the remainder of the country there is a north–south divide with the southern half of the country having significantly lower rates.

About three quarters of cancers of the mouth are related to smoking or other tobacco use, such as chewing tobacco or using snuff. Alcohol use is also a risk factor. The risk from heavy smoking and drinking is greatly increased compared with the risk of heavy smoking or heavy alcohol consumption alone.

Some mouth tumours can be removed by surgery and treated with subsequent radiotherapy and chemotherapy. Surgery can lead to the disfigurement of the face, head and neck and may lead to difficulties in movement, chewing, swallowing and speech.

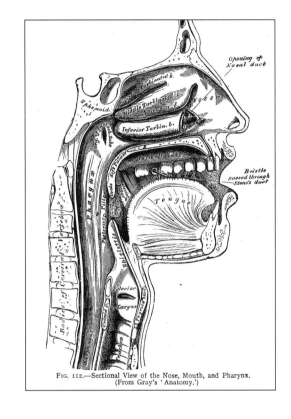

FIG. 112.—Sectional View of the Nose, Mouth, and Pharynx.
(From Gray's ' Anatomy.')

ICD-9 codes: 140-149
ICD-10 codes: C00-C14

ICD-9	ICD-9 name	% of cases	ICD-10	ICD-10 name	% of cases
141	Malignant neoplasm of tongue	22.0	C02	Malignant neoplasm of other and unspecified parts of tongue	23.3
142	Malignant neoplasm of major salivary glands	9.5	C07	Malignant neoplasm of parotid gland	7.3
143	Malignant neoplasm of gum	5.5			
144	Malignant neoplasm of floor of mouth	6.1			
145	Malignant neoplasm of other and unspecified parts of mouth	12.4	C06	Malignant neoplasm of other and unspecified parts of mouth	12.0
146	Malignant neoplasm of oropharynx	12.5	C09	Malignant neoplasm of tonsil	9.6
			C10	Malignant neoplasm of oropharynx	6.8
147	Malignant neoplasm of nasopharynx	7.7	C11	Malignant neoplasm of nasopharynx	5.8
148	Malignant neoplasm of hypopharynx	11.5	C13	Malignant neoplasm of hypopharynx	5.1
149	Malignant neoplasm of other and ill-defined sites within the lip, oral cavity and pharynx	10.9	C14	Malignant neoplasm of other and ill-defined sites in the lip, oral cavity and pharynx	9.9
	Other causes in group	1.9		Other causes in group	20.2
		100.0			100.0

MAP 60   CANCER OF THE MOUTH

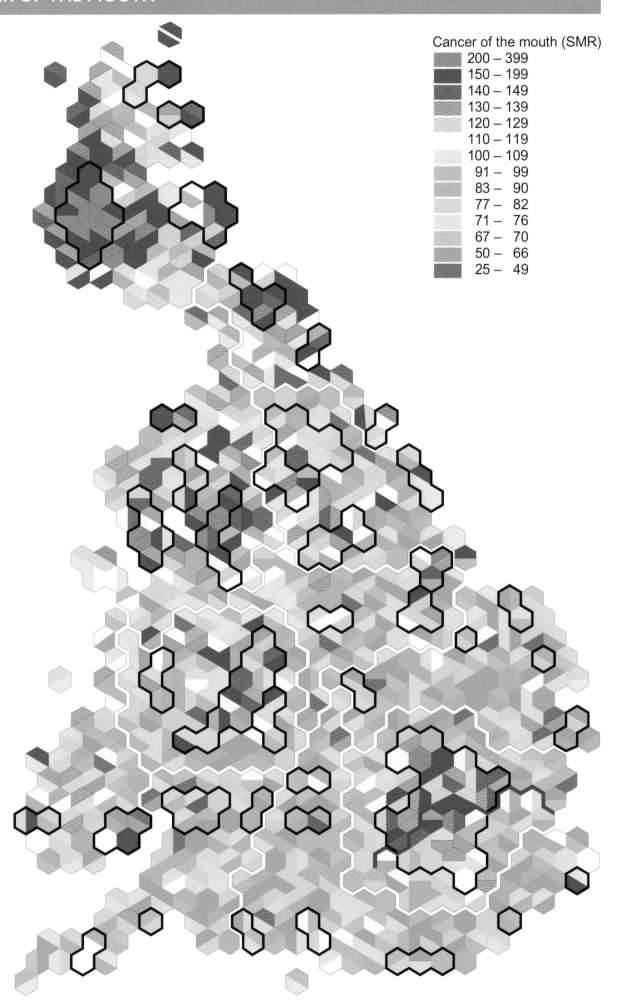

Cancer of the mouth (SMR)
- 200 – 399
- 150 – 199
- 140 – 149
- 130 – 139
- 120 – 129
- 110 – 119
- 100 – 109
- 91 – 99
- 83 – 90
- 77 – 82
- 71 – 76
- 67 – 70
- 50 – 66
- 25 – 49

62   BREAST CANCER

332,843 cases

2.24% of all deaths

average age = 68.3

male:female ratio = 1:99

Breast cancer is a sub-category of all cancers (see Map 7). Breast cancer accounts for 9% of all cancer deaths. It is the most common specific cause of death of women between ages 30 and 54.

See also Map 53 Cervical cancer, Map 59 Ovarian cancer and Map 76 Other uterine cancer.

For females, the north of England and east of Scotland tend to have lower rates than the remainder of Britain. There is little apparent geographical pattern to male breast cancer (which is much rarer).

Breast cancer is the most common cancer in women in the UK and will affect one in nine women in their lifetime. Risk factors include age (higher age leading to higher risk), early age at menarche, late age at first birth, a lower number of (or no) full-term pregnancies, short duration of (or no) breast-feeding and late age at menopause. The oral contraceptive pill and hormone replacement therapy have also been linked to breast cancer. A family history of breast cancer increases a woman's chances of having the disease herself. Being overweight or obese is one of the few modifiable risk factors; physical activity can have a protective effect.

Unlike many other cancers, breast cancer has a higher incidence in higher social classes. This is likely to reflect reproductive history and early life nutrition. However, survival rates are better for the higher social classes. The key to successful treatment of breast cancer is early diagnosis.

Approximately 1% of breast cancer deaths are of males. These are most likely to occur in males over the age of 60; men with several close family members who have had breast cancer are at a higher risk themselves. Only females are shown on the age–sex bar chart.

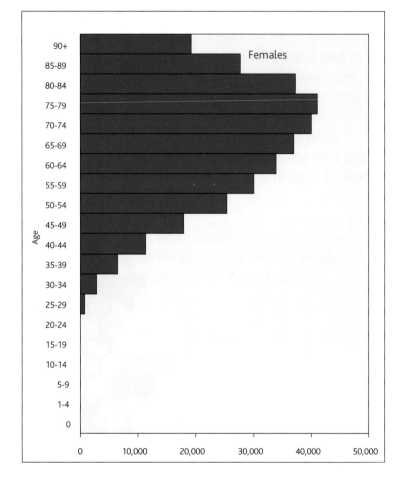

The first wife of Beatle Paul McCartney, photographer Linda McCartney, and amateur athlete and charity fundraiser Jane Tomlinson died of breast cancer.

ICD-9 codes: 174-175
ICD-10 codes: C50

ICD-9	ICD-9 name	% of cases	ICD-10	ICD-10 name	% of cases
174	Malignant neoplasm of female breast	99.4	C50	Malignant neoplasm of breast	100.0
175	Malignant neoplasm of male breast	0.6			
		100.0			100.0

MAP 62A (FEMALES) 62B (MALES)   BREAST CANCER

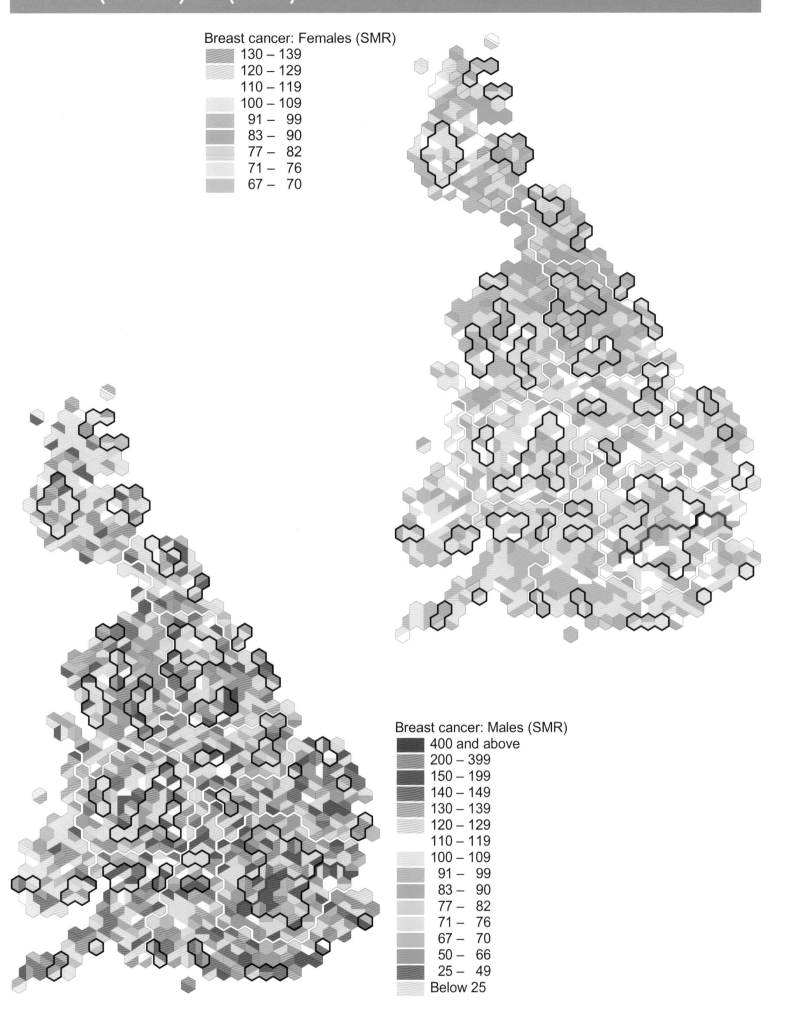

Breast cancer: Females (SMR)
- 130 – 139
- 120 – 129
- 110 – 119
- 100 – 109
- 91 – 99
- 83 – 90
- 77 – 82
- 71 – 76
- 67 – 70

Breast cancer: Males (SMR)
- 400 and above
- 200 – 399
- 150 – 199
- 140 – 149
- 130 – 139
- 120 – 129
- 110 – 119
- 100 – 109
- 91 – 99
- 83 – 90
- 77 – 82
- 71 – 76
- 67 – 70
- 50 – 66
- 25 – 49
- Below 25

63 BRONCHITIS

This is a respiratory disease and a sub-category of all respiratory deaths (see Map 10).

See also Map 55 Asthma, Map 88 Chronic lower respiratory diseases, Map 94 Industrial lung diseases, Map 97 Other respiratory disorders, Map 102 Influenza and Map 105 Pneumonia.

14,341 cases

0.10% of all deaths

average age = 68.4

male:female ratio = 41:59

Generally, the old industrial north of England tends to have the higher rates. There are also clusters of high SMRs in and around Nottingham, Scarborough, Doncaster, Hove, Hastings and Southend. The triangular cluster of rates over four times the national average in the centre of the map is Derby, Ashfield and Mansfield, where in past decades many women worked in textile mills while the men were often miners.

Bronchitis is infection in the bronchi, the airways of the lung, leading them to become inflamed and irritated. It is common in winter and often develops following a cold or flu. The main symptom is a cough that may produce a yellowy grey mucus.

Smokers are more likely to contract bronchitis. People working with grains or textiles are also more likely to develop it. Coal dust can also irritate the airways.

Babies are at a greater risk from infections in their first year of life. Acute bronchiolitis is the commonest lower respiratory infection of infancy. The risk is higher if there is smoking in the home. Babies under six months old are particularly vulnerable, but probably less so if breast fed.

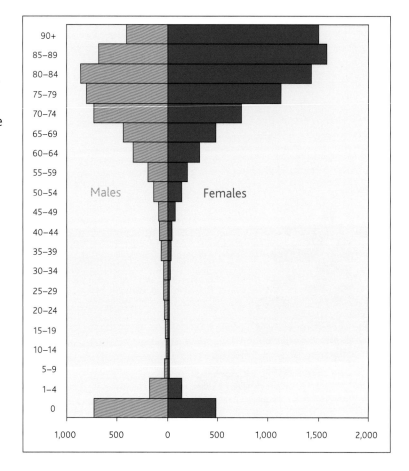

ICD-9 codes: 466
ICD-10 codes: J20-J21

ICD-9	ICD-9 name	% of cases	ICD-10	ICD-10 name	% of cases
466	Acute bronchitis and bronchiolitis	100.0	J20	Acute bronchitis	93.7
			J21	Acute bronchiolitis	6.3
		100.0			100.0

MAP 63   BRONCHITIS

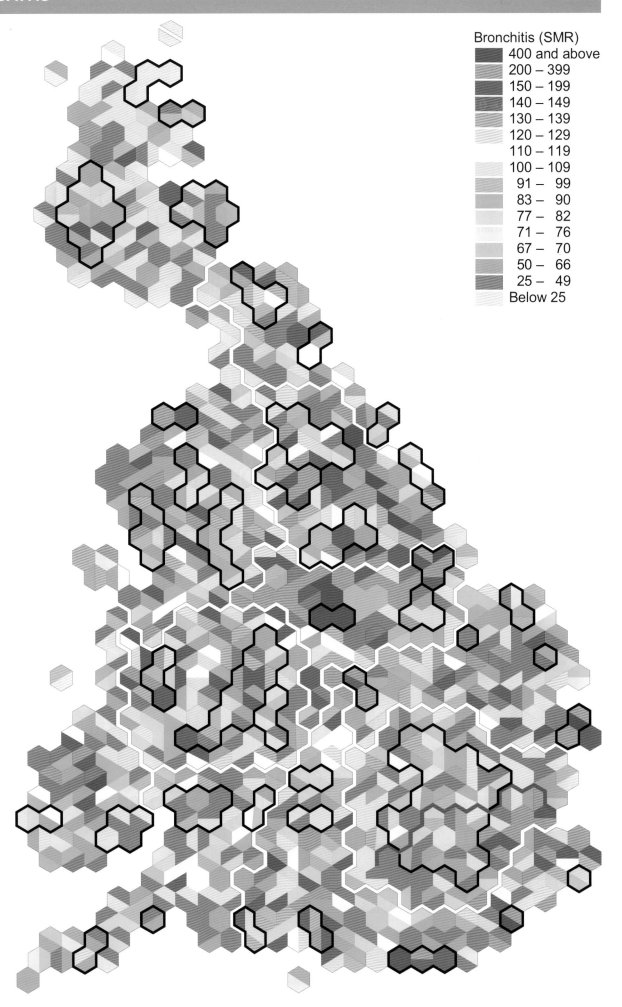

Bronchitis (SMR)
- 400 and above
- 200 – 399
- 150 – 199
- 140 – 149
- 130 – 139
- 120 – 129
- 110 – 119
- 100 – 109
- 91 – 99
- 83 – 90
- 77 – 82
- 71 – 76
- 67 – 70
- 50 – 66
- 25 – 49
- Below 25

65 LARYNGEAL CANCER

This is a form of cancer (see Map 7 All cancer deaths) affecting the larynx, which is also known as the voicebox.

See also Map 60 Cancer of the mouth, Map 68 Lung cancer and Map 71 Cancer of gullet.

21,349 cases

0.14% of all deaths

average age = 69.4

male:female ratio = 79:21

This is probably a map of smoking, drinking and poverty. The highest rates of laryngeal cancer are found in and around Glasgow, in the north west, along the north east coast and in London, followed by the West Midlands and south Wales.

The risk of lanrygeal cancer, like cancer of the mouth, is greatly increased by smoking and alcohol consumption, particularly spirits. When combined these two risk factors have a synergistic effect.

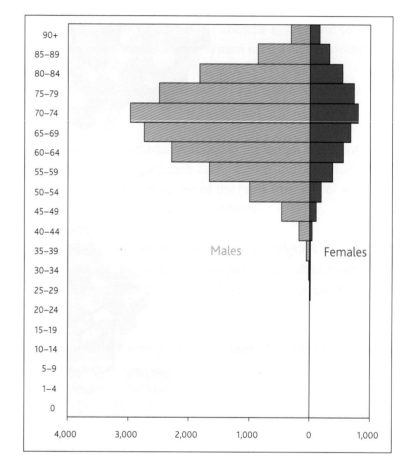

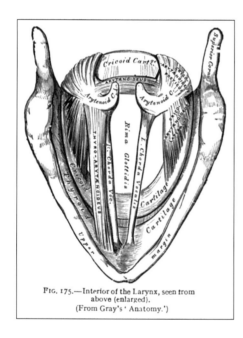

Fig. 175.—Interior of the Larynx, seen from above (enlarged). (From Gray's 'Anatomy.')

The author Evan Hunter (who also wrote as Ed McBain) died of cancer of the larynx.

Laryngeal cancer and the surgery used to treat it commonly lead to difficulty speaking and breathing. A breathing stoma is a hole in the neck that is used for breathing when the larynx has been removed by surgery or is swollen from the effects of radiotherapy.

ICD-9 codes: 161
ICD-10 codes: C32

ICD-9	ICD-9 name	% of cases	ICD-10	ICD-10 name	% of cases
161	Malignant neoplasm of larynx	100.0	C32	Malignant neoplasm of larynx	100.0
		100.0			100.0

MAP 65   LARYNGEAL CANCER

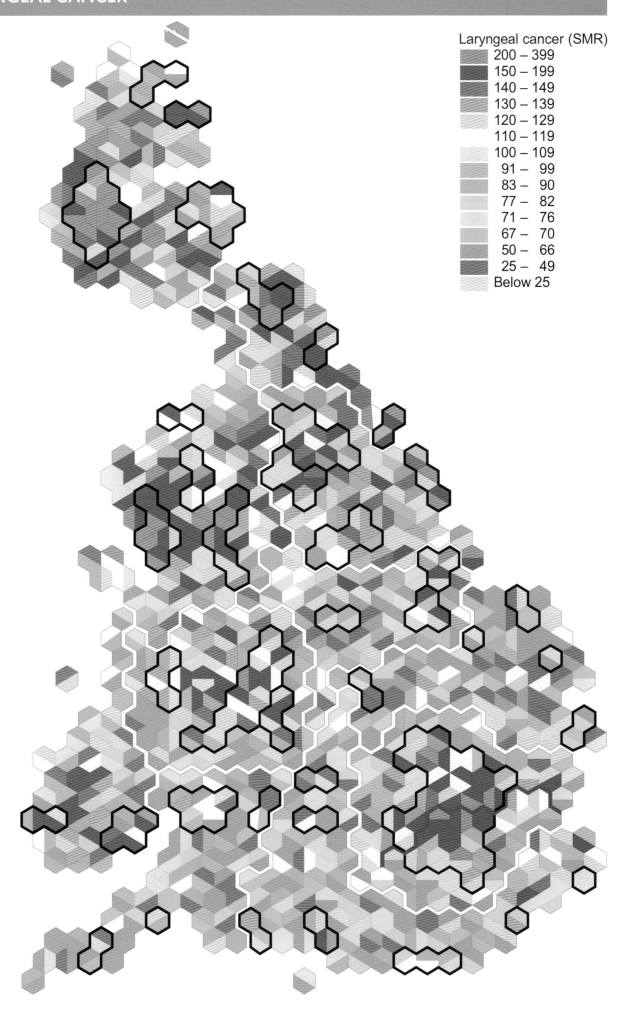

Laryngeal cancer (SMR)
- 200 – 399
- 150 – 199
- 140 – 149
- 130 – 139
- 120 – 129
- 110 – 119
- 100 – 109
- 91 – 99
- 83 – 90
- 77 – 82
- 71 – 76
- 67 – 70
- 50 – 66
- 25 – 49
- Below 25

66 TUBERCULOSIS INFECTIONS

This category includes various forms of tuberculosis, and is a sub-category of All deaths due to infections (see Map 6).

15,150 cases

0.10% of all deaths

average age = 69.6

male:female ratio = 61:39

Tuberculosis (TB) is transmitted by infectious droplets when an infected person coughs or sneezes and occasionally by unpasteurised milk from infected cows. It is linked with poverty and living in overcrowded conditions. Many cases of TB in England and Wales are also linked with recent immigrant communities; this is less the case in Scotland. The map shows very high SMRs in Glasgow, London, Birmingham and the Greater Manchester area.

CONSUMPTION: SUITABLE DAYTIME ACTIVITIES
A consumptive patient who is kept continuously in bed should not be allowed to sleep during the day, or a restless night will ensue. Knitting and reading are both suitable day-time occupations provided the patient is well enough to sit up in bed

TB is an infection caused by mycobacteria. It most commonly attacks the lungs (known as respiratory or pulmonary tuberculosis) but can also affect other organs such as the central nervous system, the lymphatic system, the circulatory system, the bones, joints and even the skin. Symptoms include chest pain, a prolonged cough and coughing up blood.

Children who catch TB are often not ill with it and become resistant to it. Adults with HIV are at much greater risk of catching TB and much harder to treat.

TB is now usually curable with antibiotics which must be taken for at least six months. Before TB could be treated in this way, in the early twentieth century, people who had the infection were commonly sent to sanatoria for many months and sometimes years, where they were treated with a regime of fresh air and rest. Some strains resistant to all antibiotics are now occurring.

TB is a disease that has a particular association with literature and the Romantic period, with poet John Keats (1795–1821) being the most notorious literary victim of TB and the epitome of the young, beautiful, doomed poet.

ICD-9 codes: 010-018, 137

ICD-10 codes: A16-A19, B90

ICD-9	ICD-9 name	% of cases	ICD-10	ICD-10 name	% of cases
011	Pulmonary tuberculosis	57.7	A16	Respiratory tuberculosis, not confirmed bacteriologically or histologically	63.4
015	Tuberculosis of bones and joints	5.0	A18	Tuberculosis of other organs	8.7
018	Miliary tuberculosis	6.3	A19	Miliary tuberculosis	7.7
137	Late effects of tuberculosis	25.2	B90	Sequelae of tuberculosis	16.8
	Other causes in group	5.8		Other causes in group	3.4
		100.0			100.0

MAP 66 TUBERCULOSIS INFECTIONS

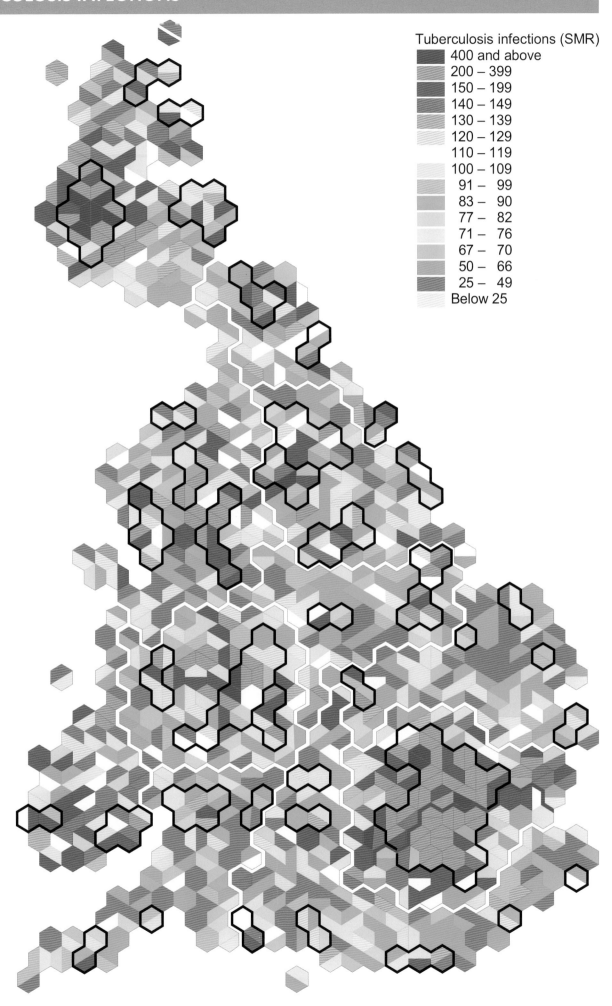

Tuberculosis infections (SMR)
- 400 and above
- 200 – 399
- 150 – 199
- 140 – 149
- 130 – 139
- 120 – 129
- 110 – 119
- 100 – 109
- 91 – 99
- 83 – 90
- 77 – 82
- 71 – 76
- 67 – 70
- 50 – 66
- 25 – 49
- Below 25

67 CANCER OF THE LIVER

This is a sub-category of All cancer deaths (see Map 7). It contains primary liver cancers, that is, when cancer starts in the liver itself. Many other primary cancers can spread to cause secondary tumours in the liver, but are not included here.

See also Map 44 Hepatitis and Map 47 Chronic liver disease.

43,207 cases

0.29% of all deaths

average age = 70.1

male:female ratio = 58:42

Males and females are mapped separately as the geographical patterns are different. For males the highest rates are found in Scotland, particularly Glasgow, Inner London, Tyneside and Liverpool; urban areas tend to have higher rates than rural. Females have the highest rates in Glasgow, and also show a similar rural–urban divide.

Primary liver cancer is a relatively rare form of cancer and is cancer in the liver itself or the bile ducts that connect the liver to the small bowel. Cancer in the liver develops mainly in people who have cirrhosis of the liver (although only a small proportion of people with cirrhosis will develop cancer of the liver). Cirrhosis can be caused by infection (for example, Hepatitis B or C) or by heavy alcohol consumption.

The author Jorge Luis Borges died of liver cancer.

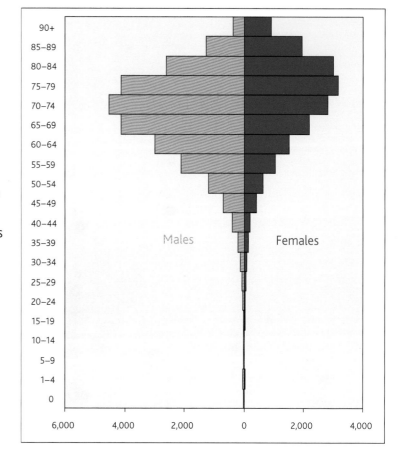

ICD-9 codes: 155
ICD-10 codes: C22

ICD-9	ICD-9 name	% of cases	ICD-10	ICD-10 name	% of cases
155	Malignant neoplasm of liver and intrahepatic bile ducts	100.0	C22	Malignant neoplasm of liver and intrahepatic bile ducts	100.0
		100.0			100.0

MAP 67A (FEMALES) 67B (MALES)   CANCER OF THE LIVER

Cancer of the liver: Females (SMR)

- 200 – 399
- 150 – 199
- 140 – 149
- 130 – 139
- 120 – 129
- 110 – 119
- 100 – 109
- 91 – 99
- 83 – 90
- 77 – 82
- 71 – 76
- 67 – 70
- 50 – 66
- 25 – 49
- Below 25

Cancer of the liver: Males (SMR)

- 200 – 399
- 150 – 199
- 140 – 149
- 130 – 139
- 120 – 129
- 110 – 119
- 100 – 109
- 91 – 99
- 83 – 90
- 77 – 82
- 71 – 76
- 67 – 70
- 50 – 66
- 25 – 49
- Below 25

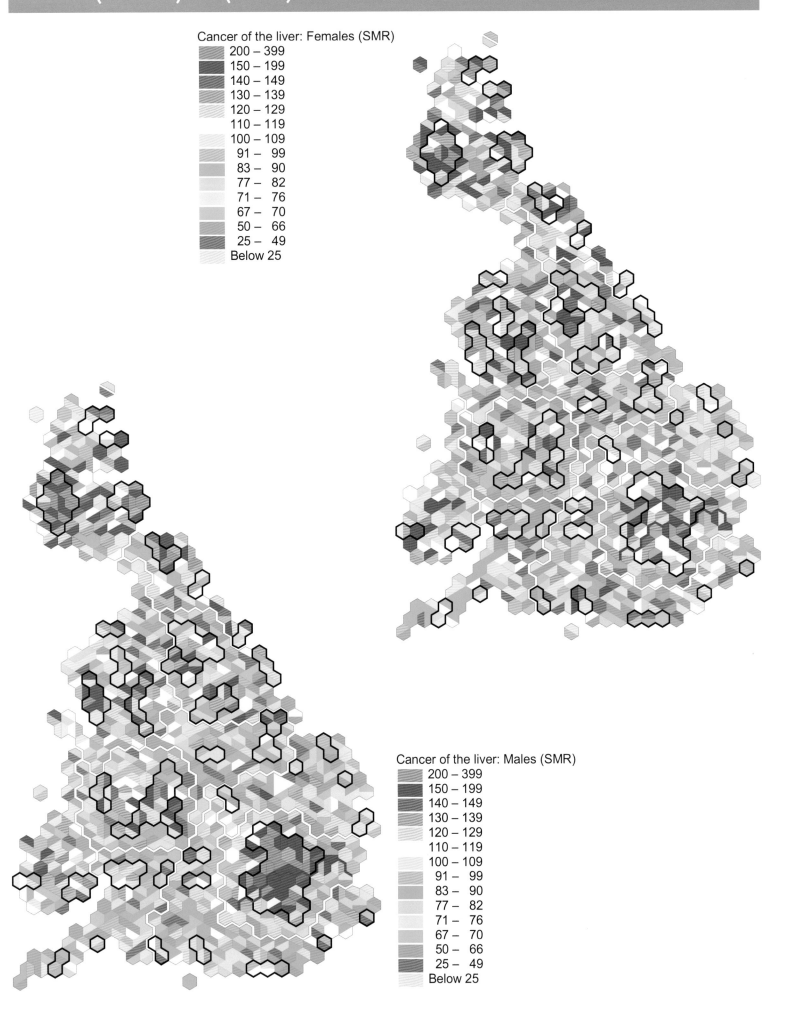

68 LUNG CANCER

This category is a sub-category of All cancer deaths (see Map 7). Lung cancer is the second most common specific cause of death of men aged between 45 and 74 after heart disease. It is the third most common cause for women aged 50–74.

See also Map 61 Other neoplasms.

872,127 cases

5.87% of all deaths

average age = 70.5

male:female ratio = 67:33

Smoking is strongly linked to deprivation. The map shows a north–south gradient with lower rates in the south. Scotland, and particularly Glasgow, has the highest rates; Scotland also has the highest smoking rates. Clusters are found in Liverpool and Manchester, in Tyneside and along the north east coast, and in central London. Within central London, the neighbourhoods covering the cities of Westminster and London, and Kensington and Chelsea – more affluent areas – have lower rates than their neighbours. The maps for male and female deaths are similar, except for higher rates for men in the West Midlands.

This category includes cancer of the lung and the bronchi, the airways of the lungs. It accounts for more than one in 20 of all deaths in the period covered in this atlas (1981 to 2004 inclusive).

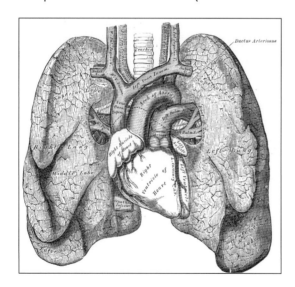

The musicians George Melly and George Harrison died of lung cancer.

Most lung cancer is caused by smoking. Lung cancer has been more common in men as traditionally they have had higher rates of smoking. However, as rates of smoking in women increased so did their rates of lung cancer.

Lung cancer is often diagnosed at an advanced stage of disease. It is one of the most difficult cancers to treat and has one of the lowest survival outcomes of any form of cancer.

ICD-9 codes: 162
ICD-10 codes: C33-C34

ICD-9	ICD-9 name	% of cases	ICD-10	ICD-10 name	% of cases
162	Malignant neoplasm of trachea, bronchus and lung	100.0	C34	Malignant neoplasm of bronchus and lung	99.9
				Other causes in group	0.1
		100.0			100.0

MAP 68   LUNG CANCER

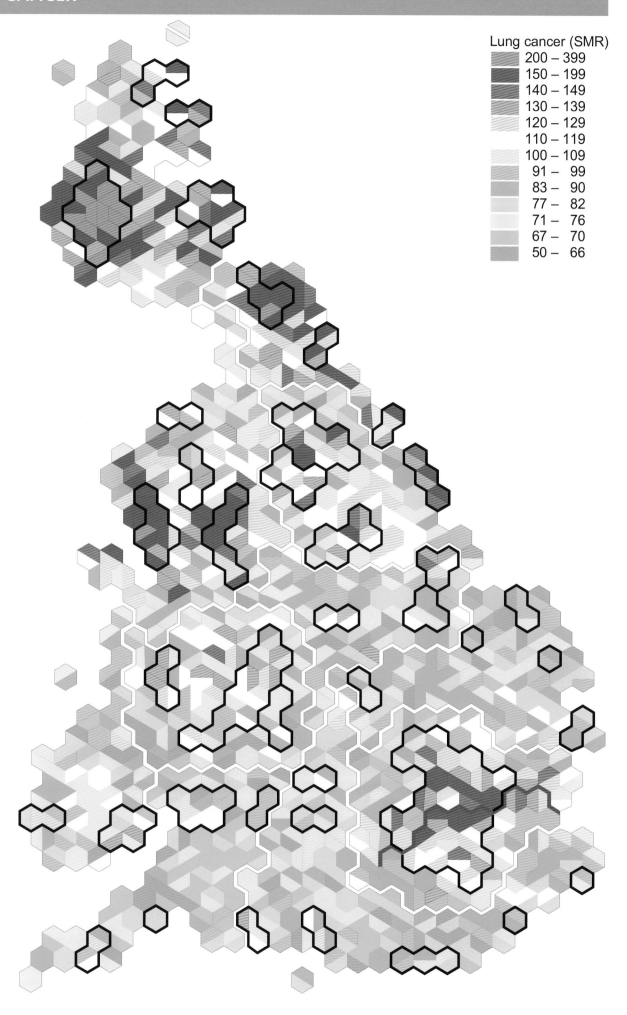

Lung cancer (SMR)
	200 – 399
	150 – 199
	140 – 149
	130 – 139
	120 – 129
	110 – 119
	100 – 109
	91 – 99
	83 – 90
	77 – 82
	71 – 76
	67 – 70
	50 – 66

69   DURING SURGERY, MEDICAL CARE

This is an external cause of death.

See also Map 52 Other external causes, which includes complications relating to surgery and medical care.

8,662 cases

0.06% of all deaths

average age = 70.7

male:female ratio = 48:52

The highest rates are found in Scotland. Whether this is an artefact of different ICD coding of hospital deaths is not known. However, given that Scotland tends to have poorer health than the remainder of Britain, it is likely that surgical outcomes could well be poorer. Scotland also had far more hospital beds and hence more surgery taking place over the period studied here than other areas of Britain. Other clusters of high rates are found in Tyneside, around Birmingham and Manchester.

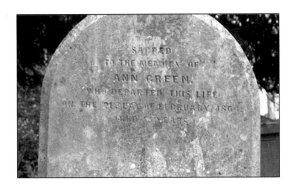

This is a relatively rare cause of death (on average, one per day) that is evenly distributed among men and women. Many of the cases are due to unavoidable risks of the particular surgery undertaken. Some of the cases are due to errors by surgeons, anaesthetists and other medical personnel. Others can be due to adverse reactions to drug treatment. Much depends, however, on how sick the patient was at the time – a fitter, healthier patient being likely to have better survival chances than a very frail one. Additionally, the complexity of the surgery itself is also a factor; emergency surgery carries a higher risk than elective.

The dramatic increase in people undergoing cosmetic surgery may see rates rise in the future, and see the average age decrease.

Stella Obasanjo, the first lady of Nigeria, and Olivia Goldsmith, author of The First Wives Club, *both died while undergoing cosmetic surgery.*

ICD-9 codes: E870-E876, E878-E879
ICD-10 codes: Y60-Y63, Y65, Y83-Y84, Y88

ICD-9	ICD-9 name	% of cases	ICD-10	ICD-10 name	% of cases
E870	Accidental cut, puncture, perforation or haemorrhage during medical care	15.7	Y60	Unintentional cut, puncture, perforation or haemorrhage during surgical and medical care	8.0
E878	Surgical operation and other surgical procedures as the cause of abnormal reaction of patient, or of later complication, without mention of misadventure at the time of operation	71.1	Y83	Surgical operation and other surgical procedures as the cause of abnormal reaction of the patient, or of later complication, without mention of misadventure at the time of the procedure	77.7
E879	Other procedures, without mention of misadventure at the time of procedure, as the cause of abnormal reaction of patient, or of later complication	9.6	Y84	Other medical procedures as the cause of abnormal reaction of the patient, or of later complication, without mention of misadventure at the time of the procedure	12.7
	Other causes in group	3.6		Other causes in group	1.6
		100.0			100.0

MAP 69   DURING SURGERY, MEDICAL CARE

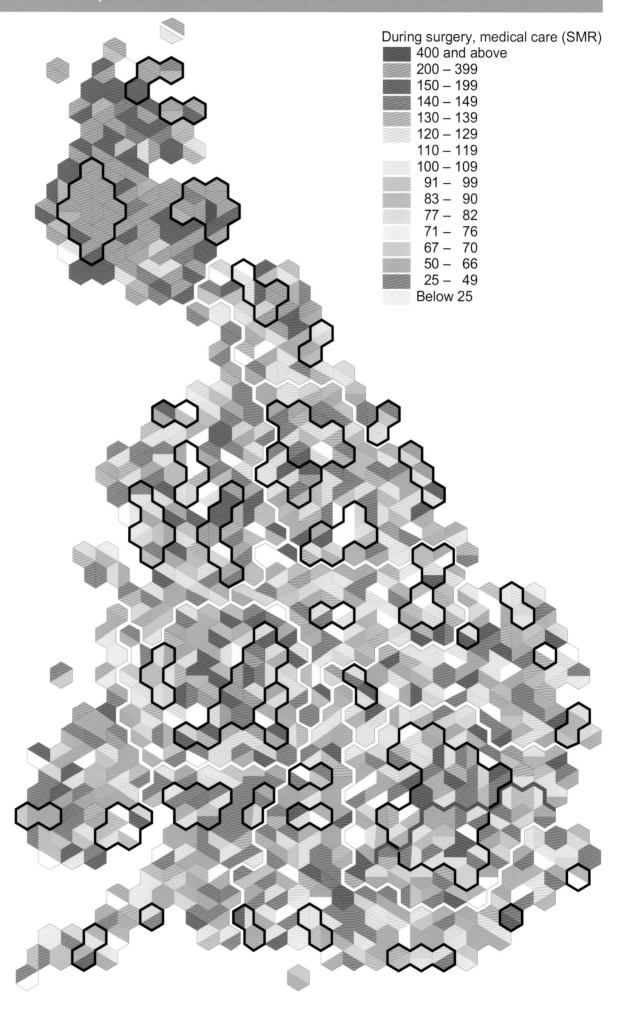

During surgery, medical care (SMR)

- 400 and above
- 200 – 399
- 150 – 199
- 140 – 149
- 130 – 139
- 120 – 129
- 110 – 119
- 100 – 109
- 91 – 99
- 83 – 90
- 77 – 82
- 71 – 76
- 67 – 70
- 50 – 66
- 25 – 49
- Below 25

70 OTHER NERVOUS DISORDERS

This category contains a range of diseases affecting the central nervous system.

See also Map 48 Multiple sclerosis and Map 56 Motor neurone disease.

117,082 cases

0.79% of all deaths

average age = 71.7

male:female ratio = 41:59

Scotland, rural north west England and the south of England generally have low rates of death from other nervous disorders. Higher rates are found in the remainder of the north of England, the Midlands and Wales. Particular clusters are found around Cardiff and Yorkshire.

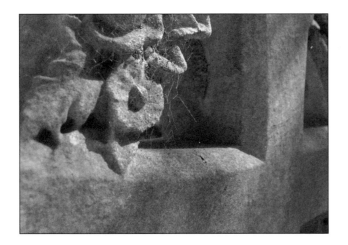

Recently (ICD-10) two thirds of the deaths in this category have been attributed to Alzheimer's disease; over the 24-year period studied here, 41% of the deaths in this category were attributed to Alzheimer's. It is progressive and terminal. The disease usually starts with mild cognitive impairment, such as short-term memory loss. The disease is named after a German psychiatrist who first identified it in 1901. Before ICD-10 it was not often recorded as the primary cause of death, but just as a contributory factor.

Other causes in this group include encephalitis, intracranial and intraspinal abscess and granuloma, Huntington's disease, infantile cerebral palsy, hemiplegia, paraplegia and tetraplegia.

Prime MInister Harold Wilson, US President Ronald Reagan and novelist Iris Murdoch had Alzheimer's disease; folk musician Woody Guthrie died of Huntington's disease.

ICD-9 codes: 323-326, 330-331, 333-334, 336-337, 341-344, 346-366, 369-370, 372, 374-378, 380-386, 388-389
ICD-10 codes: E75.0-E75.1, E75.4, F84.2, G04, G06, G08-G11, G21.0, G23-G25, G30-G31, G36-G37, G47.4, G50-G52, G54, G57-G58, G60-G62, G64, G70.0, G70.8-G70.9, G71-G72, G80-G83, G90-G92, G93.0-G93.2, G93.4-G93.9, G95-G96, G98, H05, H20, H25-H26, H34-H35, H40, H44, H47, H49, H51-H52, H54, H60-H61, H66, H70-H72, H74, H81, H91

ICD-9	ICD-9 name	% of cases	ICD-10	ICD-10 name	% of cases
331	Other cerebral degenerations	43.4	G30	Alzheimer's disease	67.2
342	Hemiplegia	20.8			
359	Muscular dystrophies and other myopathies	5.5			
	Other causes in group	30.3		Other causes in group	32.8
		100.0			100.0

MAP 70   OTHER NERVOUS DISORDERS

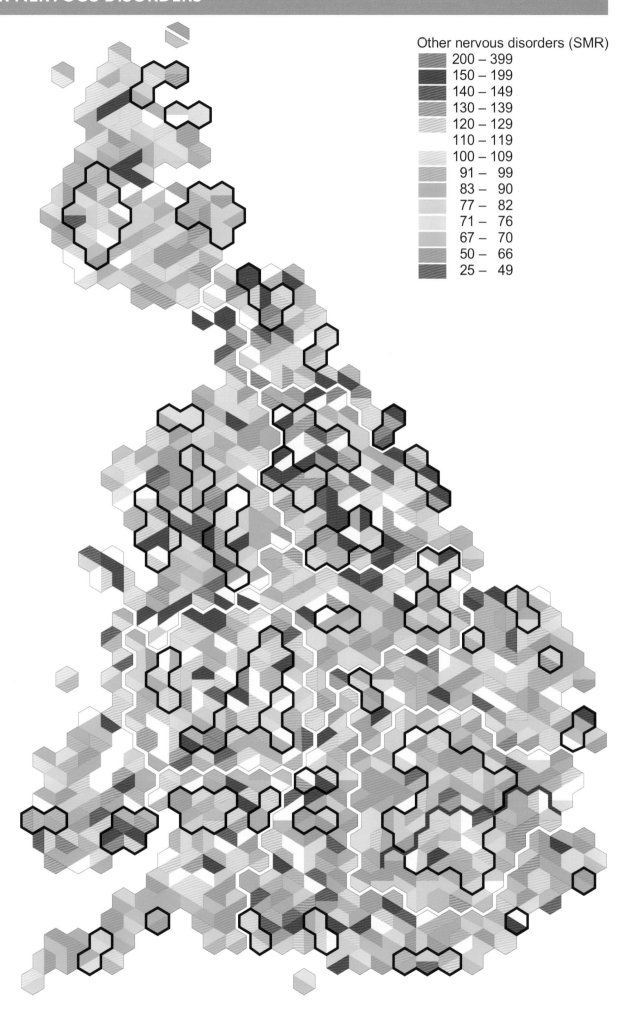

Other nervous disorders (SMR)

	200 – 399
	150 – 199
	140 – 149
	130 – 139
	120 – 129
	110 – 119
	100 – 109
	91 – 99
	83 – 90
	77 – 82
	71 – 76
	67 – 70
	50 – 66
	25 – 49

71   CANCER OF GULLET

This is a subcategory of All cancer deaths (see Map 7). Cancer of gullet is also known as oesophageal cancer.

See also Map 60 Cancer of the mouth, and Map 65 Laryngeal cancer.

143,534 cases

0.97% of all deaths

average age = 71.7

male:female ratio = 61:39

There is an east–west divide across England and Wales, with the north west and the West Midlands having higher rates than the remainder of England and almost all of Wales. The highest rates are found in Scotland, probably partly reflecting the higher smoking and drinking rates there for the population in the past.

The gullet, also known as the oesophagus or foodpipe, is a tube that connects the mouth to the stomach. A tumour in the gullet can lead to difficulty swallowing (dysphagia) and pain when swallowing (odynophagia). Smaller tumours can be removed by surgery whereas larger ones are not curable.

Increased risk of cancer of the gullet has been found to be linked to factors such as heredity, tobacco smoking, alcohol, gastroesophageal reflux disease, human papillomavirus and obesity.

A chain smoker both on and off screen, Humphrey Bogart died from oesophageal cancer.

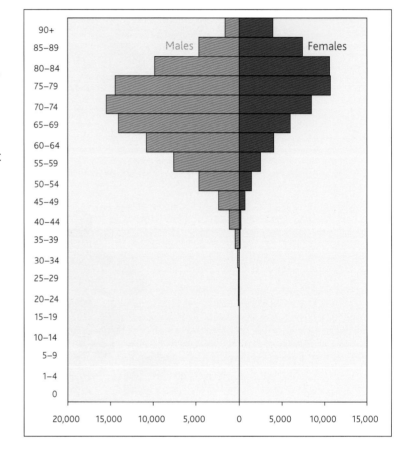

ICD-9 codes: 150
ICD-10 codes: C15

ICD-9	ICD-9 name	% of cases	ICD-10	ICD-10 name	% of cases
150	Malignant neoplasm of oesophagus	100.0	C15	Malignant neoplasm of oesophagus	100.0
		100.0			100.0

MAP 71   CANCER OF GULLET

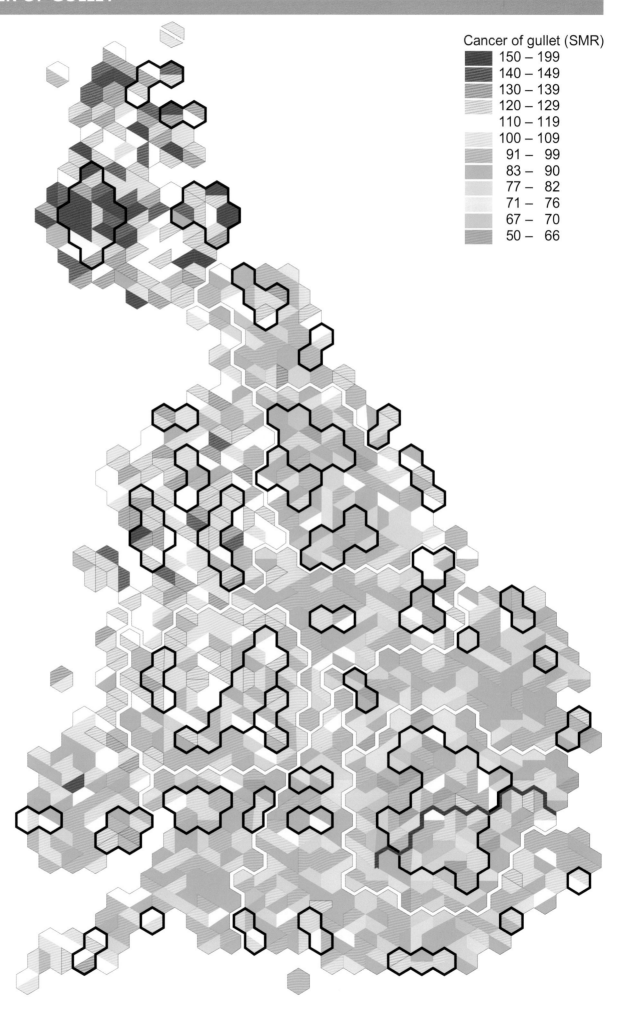

Cancer of gullet (SMR)
	150 – 199
	140 – 149
	130 – 139
	120 – 129
	110 – 119
	100 – 109
	91 – 99
	83 – 90
	77 – 82
	71 – 76
	67 – 70
	50 – 66

72 PANCREATIC CANCER

155,846 cases

1.05% of all deaths

average age = 71.9

male:female ratio = 49:51

This is a subcategory of All cancer deaths (see Map 7).

See also Map 68 Lung cancer and Map 78 Stomach cancer.

There appears to be no strong geographical pattern to rates of mortality from pancreatic cancer. The highest rates are found in the rural parts of Eilean Siar, Poplar in east London, Dyce in Aberdeen, Ladywood East in Birmingham and Middlesbrough East. Although three times as common in smokers as non-smokers, other factors must be sufficiently important for this cancer not to have a similar geographical distribution to other smoking-related cancers, such as lung cancer.

The pancreas is a large gland that is part of the digestive system. It makes digestive juices and insulin. The risk of pancreatic cancer can be increased by smoking, a diet high in sugar and fat, and long-term heavy drinking.

The early signs of pancreatic cancer can be vague – loss of appetite, sickness, general discomfort and pain in the abdominal area – and because the pancreas is deep within the body it can be difficult to make a diagnosis. Due to the fact that there are often no early indications of the disease that are noticeable to the sufferer it is often diagnosed at an advanced stage resulting in a poor prognosis.

Singer Syd Barrett, actress Joan Crawford, poet Cecil Day-Lewis, philosopher Jacques Derrida, actor Rex Harrison, journalist Miles Kington, opera singer Luciano Pavarotti and dramatist Dennis Potter all died from this cause of death.

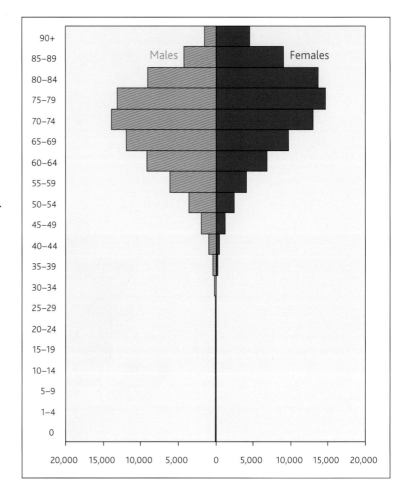

ICD-9 codes: 157

ICD-10 codes: C25

ICD-9	ICD-9 name	% of cases	ICD-10	ICD-10 name	% of cases
157	Malignant neoplasm of pancreas	100.0	C25	Malignant neoplasm of pancreas	100.0
		100.0			100.0

MAP 72   PANCREATIC CANCER

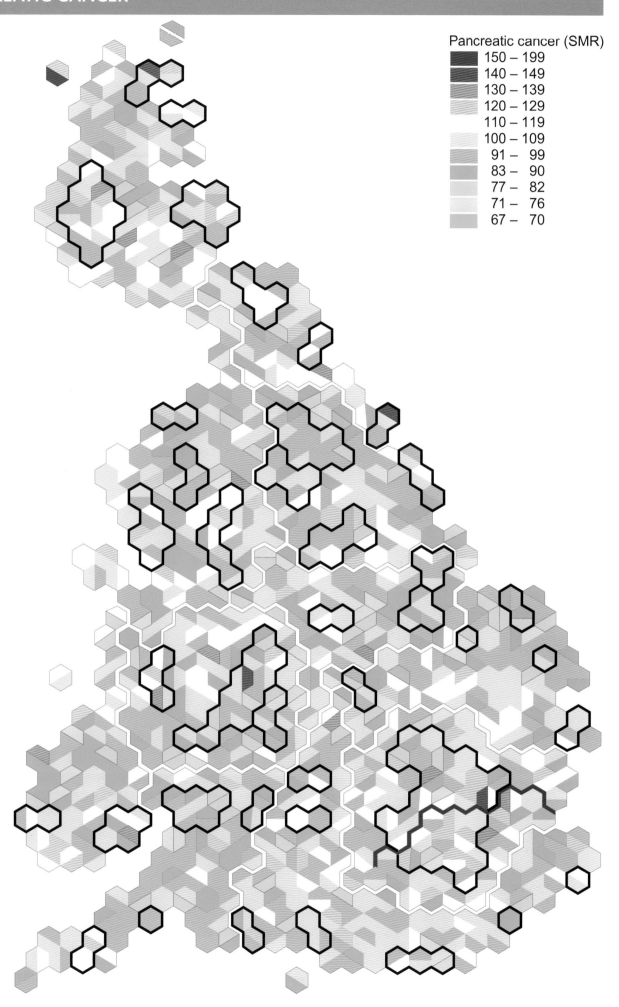

Pancreatic cancer (SMR)
- 150 – 199
- 140 – 149
- 130 – 139
- 120 – 129
- 110 – 119
- 100 – 109
- 91 – 99
- 83 – 90
- 77 – 82
- 71 – 76
- 67 – 70

73 SEPTICAEMIA

Septicaemia, commonly known as blood poisoning, is a bacterial infection of the blood.

See also Map 23 Meningitis.

29,538 cases

0.19% of all deaths

average age = 72.5

male:female ratio = 44:56

Scotland stands out as having high rates, particularly in and around Glasgow. Tyneside, the south Wales valleys, Manchester, the Portsmouth and Southampton area, Grimsby and Birmingham are all areas with high rates. Many of these are areas that have high rates of limiting long-term illness. However, rates are not especially high in Liverpool, Sheffield, Bradford and Leeds, nor in Middlesbrough, most of Stoke and Cardiff. Thus septicaemia is not simply an affliction of poorer urban areas.

Anyone can develop septicaemia, but those with weakened immune systems and pre-existing illness are more susceptible. It is often the result of another infection within the body, for instance in the lungs or kidneys, getting into the bloodstream. Older people, children, intravenous drug users and people in intensive care units are more at risk. The symptoms are high fever, violent shaking, faintness, cold and pale hands and feet, rapid and shallow breathing, restlessness, delirium, shock and loss of consciousness. If treated early enough most people make a full recovery.

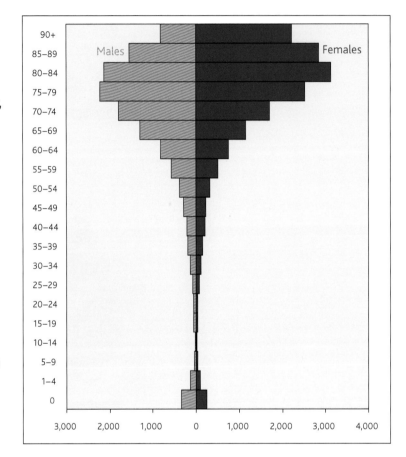

ICD-9 codes: 038

ICD-10 codes: A40-A41

ICD-9	ICD-9 name	% of cases	ICD-10	ICD-10 name	% of cases
038	Septicaemia	100.0	A40	Streptococcal septicaemia	4.6
			A41	Other septicaemia (excludes streptococcal septicaemia)	95.4
		100.0			100.0

MAP 76   OTHER UTERINE CANCER

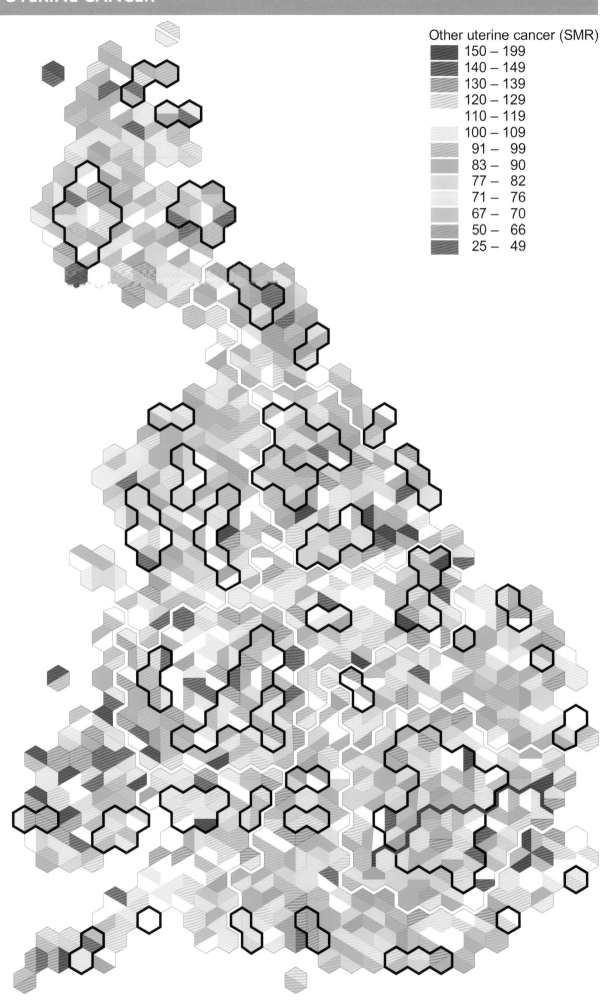

Other uterine cancer (SMR)

	150 – 199
	140 – 149
	130 – 139
	120 – 129
	110 – 119
	100 – 109
	91 – 99
	83 – 90
	77 – 82
	71 – 76
	67 – 70
	50 – 66
	25 – 49

77 UNSPECIFIED NEOPLASMS

This is a sub-category of All cancer deaths (see Map 7) that accounts for 11% of all cancers.

408,874 cases

2.76% of all deaths

average age = 73.0

male:female ratio = 49:51

The lowest rates are found in the Home Counties, rural Scotland and the south west of England. High rates tend to be found in the north, with Tyneside, Merseyside and Manchester standing out. There is a further cluster of high rates in east London.

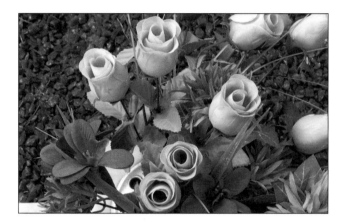

Often when diagnosis is late cancer has spread to more than one site. Diagnosis is more often late where people are less well informed of the symptoms of illness and where they generally expect to feel ill more often.

When someone has been classified as dying from 'Unspecified neoplasms' it means that no single primary site of the cancer has been noted on the death certificate. Occasionally this is because there are multiple primary sites of cancer, and it is not known which of these cancers was the cause of death. Often it is because cancer was not diagnosed until it had spread, most commonly to the liver. It may not be obvious where this secondary cancer arose from. Cancer that has spread is often incurable, and ascertaining the original site is only of academic value.

ICD-9 codes: 159, 195-196, 198-199, 235-239

ICD-10 codes: C26, C76-C80, C90.2, C97, D37-D43, D44.0-D44.1, D44.3-D44.7, D44.9, D45-D46, D47.1, D47.3, D47.7, D47.9, D48, Q85.0

ICD-9	ICD-9 name	% of cases	ICD-10	ICD-10 name	% of cases
199	Malignant neoplasm without specification of site	78.7	C80	Malignant neoplasm without specification of site	60.0
			C97	Malignant neoplasms of independent (primary) multiple sites	5.1
159	Malignant neoplasm of other and ill-defined sites within the digestive organs and peritoneum	7.6	C26	Malignant neoplasm of other and ill-defined digestive organs	11.2
			D46	Myelodysplastic syndromes	5.3
239	Neoplasm of unspecified nature	7.5			
	Other causes in group	6.2		Other causes in group	18.4
		100.0			100.0

MAP 77   UNSPECIFIED NEOPLASMS

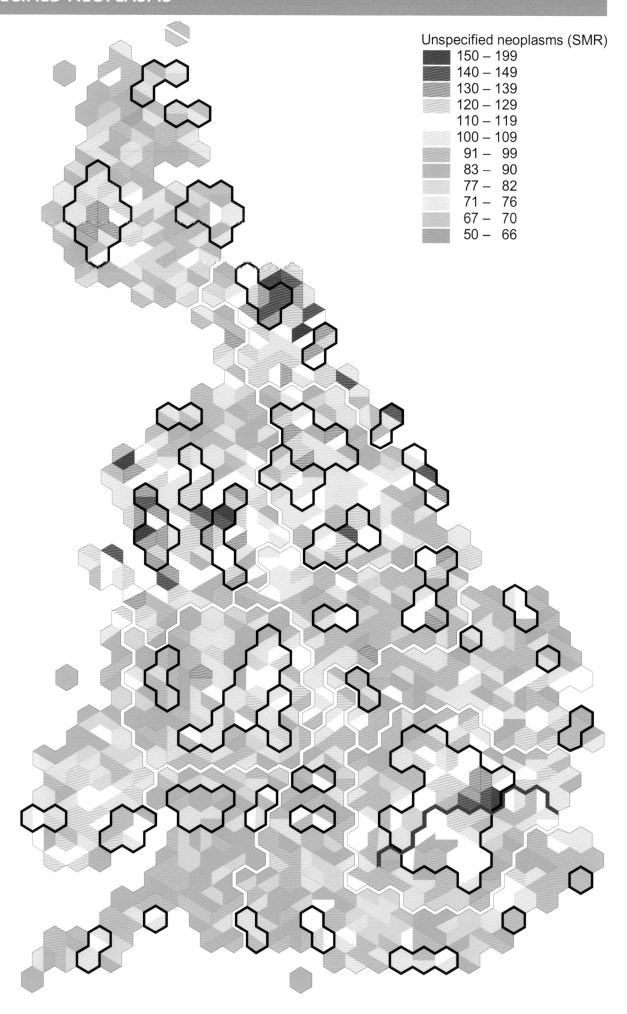

Unspecified neoplasms (SMR)
- 150 – 199
- 140 – 149
- 130 – 139
- 120 – 129
- 110 – 119
- 100 – 109
- 91 – 99
- 83 – 90
- 77 – 82
- 71 – 76
- 67 – 70
- 50 – 66

78 STOMACH CANCER

This is a subcategory of All cancer deaths (see Map 7).

The stomach is part of the digestive system. See also Map 71 Cancer of gullet, Map 72 Pancreatic cancer, Map 74 Rectal cancer and Map 79 Colon cancer.

208,452 cases

1.41% of all deaths

average age = 73.1

male:female ratio = 60:40

There is generally a north–south divide, with the area south of a line drawn from the Severn to the Wash having lower rates, apart from London. There is a cluster of particularly high rates in Stoke-on-Trent, with Glasgow, other northern urban areas and the south Wales valleys also having high rates. The correlation between poverty and dying from this form of cancer is high enough for it in many cases to mark out the poorer quarters of particular towns and cities on this map.

Stomach cancer is more common in people with poor diets and high alcohol and tobacco consumption. Rates have fallen in recent decades. This is thought to be related to falling rates of *Helicobacter pylori* (*H pylori*) infection. Changes in diet, in particular the refrigeration of food, and eating less pickled and smoked food, may also play a role. Other factors which increase the risk of stomach cancer are pernicious anaemia and atrophic gastritis (a stomach disorder).

H pylori is an infection of the stomach and duodenum that as well as causing stomach cancer can lead to gastritis, peptic ulcers and duodenitis. It was a common infection but rates have fallen for each successive birth cohort over the past several decades. Once you have the infection, untreated it usually stays with you for life, but infected people often have no symptoms before getting the conditions listed above.

High levels of *H pylori* infection have been found to be associated with living in poor socioeconomic conditions and poverty during childhood; children who live in poverty are therefore more likely to get stomach cancer later in life (see 'Introduction' in G. Davey Smith (2003) *Health inequalities: Lifecourse approaches*, Bristol: The Policy Press).

Writer Gertrude Stein, actor John Wayne, footballer and manager Brian Clough and Prime Minister Neville Chamberlain died from this cause.

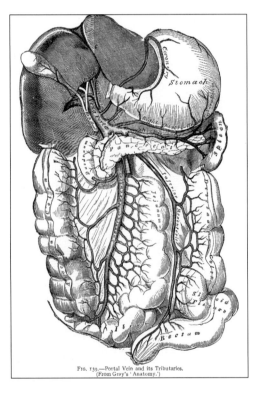

FIG. 139.—Portal Vein and its Tributaries.
(From Gray's 'Anatomy.')

ICD-9 codes: 151
ICD-10 codes: C16

ICD-9	ICD-9 name	% of cases	ICD-10	ICD-10 name	% of cases
151	Malignant neoplasm of stomach	100.0	C16	Malignant neoplasm of stomach	100.0
		100.0			100.0

MAP 78   STOMACH CANCER

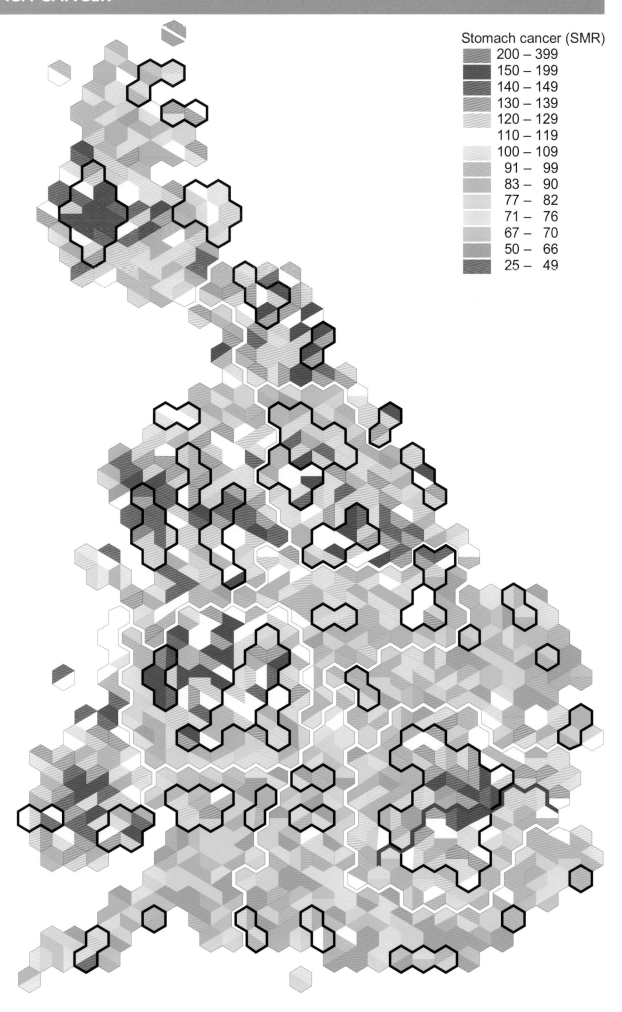

Stomach cancer (SMR)

	200 – 399
	150 – 199
	140 – 149
	130 – 139
	120 – 129
	110 – 119
	100 – 109
	91 – 99
	83 – 90
	77 – 82
	71 – 76
	67 – 70
	50 – 66
	25 – 49

79 COLON CANCER

This is a sub-category of All cancer deaths (see Map 7). The colon is part of the digestive system. Colon cancer and rectal cancer are referred to as 'colorectal cancer' or 'bowel cancer'.

See also Map 71 Cancer of gullet, Map 72 Pancreatic cancer, Map 74 Rectal cancer and Map 78 Stomach cancer.

277,820 cases

1.87% of all deaths

average age = 73.4

male:female ratio = 47:53

This map is very different from both that for rectal cancer (Map 74) and that for stomach cancer (Map 78). Rates here do not reach the extremes shown on those maps.

There is an east–west divide, with rates in the west higher than those to the east. Northern Scotland, and west Wales tend to have the higher rates, with particularly high rates found in Liverpool Riverside North, Montrose and Arbroath, and Dyce in Aberdeen.

The low rates in Yorkshire seen here are similar to the low rates also seen there for deaths from cancer of the gullet.

Colon cancer is cancer of the large bowel. It starts with the abnormal growth of cells in the lining of the bowel. Small lumps called polyps, which can also be referred to as tumours, form; they are usually benign, but can become malignant. Malignant tumours can spread to other parts of the body.

As with rectal cancer, a change in bowel habits or blood in the stool can be the first indication of disease. If diagnosed early, then bowel cancer can be cured. There is an NHS Bowel Cancer Screening programme that is offered every two years to all men and women aged 60–69. A diet high in fibre may help to prevent this type of cancer.

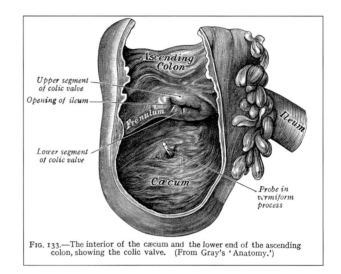

FIG. 133.—The interior of the cæcum and the lower end of the ascending colon, showing the colic valve. (From Gray's 'Anatomy.')

Israeli politician Moshe Dayan and singer songwriter Ian Dury died from this cause.

ICD-9 codes: 153
ICD-10 codes: C18

ICD-9	ICD-9 name	% of cases	ICD-10	ICD-10 name	% of cases
153	Malignant neoplasm of colon	100.0	C18	Malignant neoplasm of colon	100.0
		100.0			100.0

MAP 79   COLON CANCER

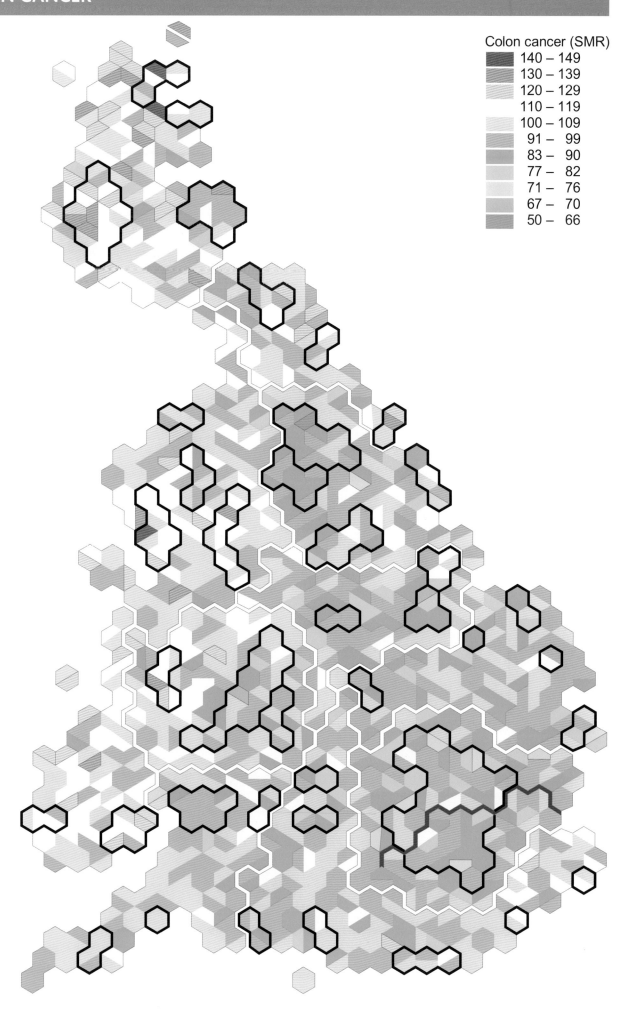

Colon cancer (SMR)
- 140 – 149
- 130 – 139
- 120 – 129
- 110 – 119
- 100 – 109
- 91 – 99
- 83 – 90
- 77 – 82
- 71 – 76
- 67 – 70
- 50 – 66

80 SIGNS AND SYMPTOMS

3,131 cases

0.02% of all deaths

average age = 74.1

male:female ratio = 36:64

The category Signs and Symptoms contains a range of disorders and diseases.

'Signs' refers to evidence of disease as perceived by a doctor; 'symptoms' refers to evidence of disease as perceived by the patient. In general this diagnosis of cause of death implies uncertainty on behalf of the person completing the death certificate.

The female map shows a cluster along the north east coast between Jarrow and Middlesbrough. Over the years that this atlas covers, an unusually high number of elderly women lived alone in the north east, often widows who had not remarried. Housing was plentiful, which also made living alone easier there – but simultaneously fewer women will have had partners who might query the diagnosis or encourage them to seek help earlier.

This group of causes of death includes symptoms, signs and abnormal test results as well as ill-defined conditions for which there is no diagnosis classification elsewhere. This could be because a person has less well-defined conditions and symptoms, or has multiple symptoms that might point to two or more diseases.

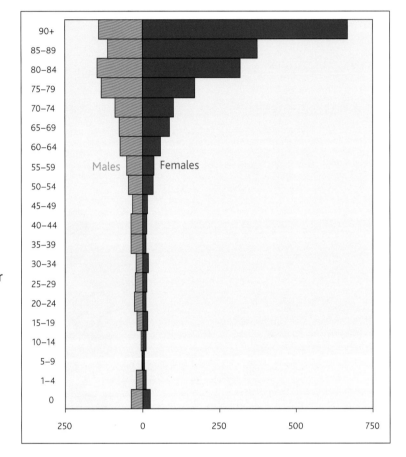

ICD-9 codes: 780-791, 793, 795-796

ICD-10 codes: E03.5, G47.3, G93.3, N23, N39.4, R02, R04-R06, R09.8, R10-R11, R13-R14, R16-R17, R19, R21, R23, R27, R39, R41.3, R41.8, R50, R53, R55-R57, R59-R60, R62-R63, R68, R73, R90-R91

ICD-9	ICD-9 name	% of cases	ICD-10	ICD-10 name	% of cases
780	General symptoms	21.8	G47.3	Sleep apnoea	7.0
			R53	Malaise and fatigue	39.5
			R68	Other general symptoms and signs	16.2
785	Symptoms involving cardiovascular system	48.3			
786	Symptoms involving respiratory system and other chest symptoms	10.2			
789	Other symptoms involving abdomen and pelvis	6.9	R19.8	Other specified symptoms and signs involving the digestive system and abdomen	14.3
	Other causes in group	12.8		Other causes in group	23.0
		100.0			100.0

MAP 80A (FEMALES) 80B (MALES)   SIGNS AND SYMPTOMS

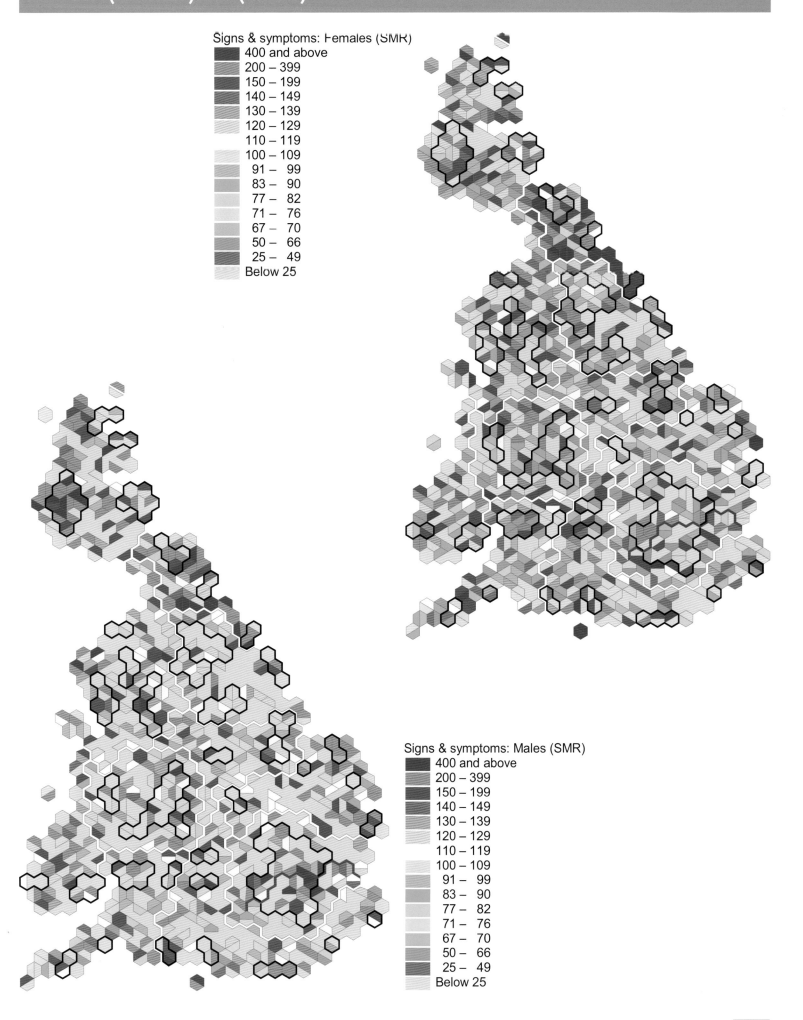

Signs & symptoms: Females (SMR)
- 400 and above
- 200 – 399
- 150 – 199
- 140 – 149
- 130 – 139
- 120 – 129
- 110 – 119
- 100 – 109
- 91 – 99
- 83 – 90
- 77 – 82
- 71 – 76
- 67 – 70
- 50 – 66
- 25 – 49
- Below 25

Signs & symptoms: Males (SMR)
- 400 and above
- 200 – 399
- 150 – 199
- 140 – 149
- 130 – 139
- 120 – 129
- 110 – 119
- 100 – 109
- 91 – 99
- 83 – 90
- 77 – 82
- 71 – 76
- 67 – 70
- 50 – 66
- 25 – 49
- Below 25

81 HYPOTHERMIA

Hypothermia is an external cause of death. See Map 5 All external deaths. The term refers to the condition where severe cold causes death.

See also Map 50 Hunger, thirst, exposure, neglect.

5,316 cases

0.04% of all deaths

average age = 74.8

male:female ratio = 44:56

Rates of death from hypothermia are low, so the map has a somewhat patchy appearance. The southern part of Inner London, Birmingham and Scottish cities record some of the highest rates; in each, males tend to have higher rates than females. These are areas where higher than average numbers of older people live alone, may not have central heating and are likely to be living in fuel poverty; both the high costs of housing in the south and the need to heat for longer in the north may be factors that influence this map's appearance.

Hypothermia is when the temperature of the body drops below normal and the metabolism and bodily functions are affected. In its most severe form, when the body temperature drops below 32^{0}C, the pulse and respiration rates decrease, major organs fail and clinical death occurs. Due to decreased cellular activity in the cold conditions, brain death will take longer to occur: a person suffering from hypothermia should not be assumed dead until they are 'warm dead'. The body needs to be brought into a warm environment to confirm mortality.

In Britain, most people who die from hypothermia are elderly people living alone, especially women, who have become cold inside their homes, rather than outside. Poverty, the cost of heating a home and substandard housing all play a part; the elderly are particularly vulnerable, hence the government's Winter Fuel Payments.

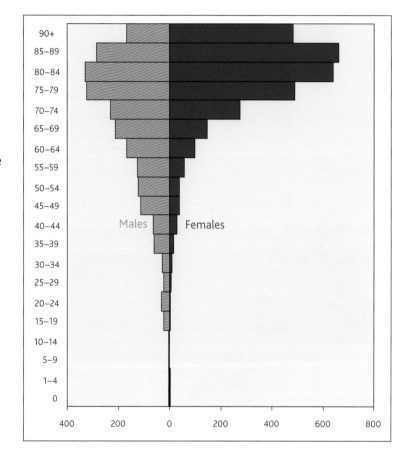

Under 65 years old, more men than women die of hypothermia. Some of these will have been living rough, some unable to get home because of being drunk, and some deaths will be from leisure activities (such as mountaineering or fell walking) that have gone badly wrong.

ICD-9 codes: E901
ICD-10 codes: W93, X31

ICD-9	ICD-9 name	% of cases	ICD-10	ICD-10 name	% of cases
E901	Excessive cold	100.0	X31	Exposure to excessive natural cold	99.0
				Other causes in group	1.0
		100.0			100.0

MAP 83 BLADDER CANCER

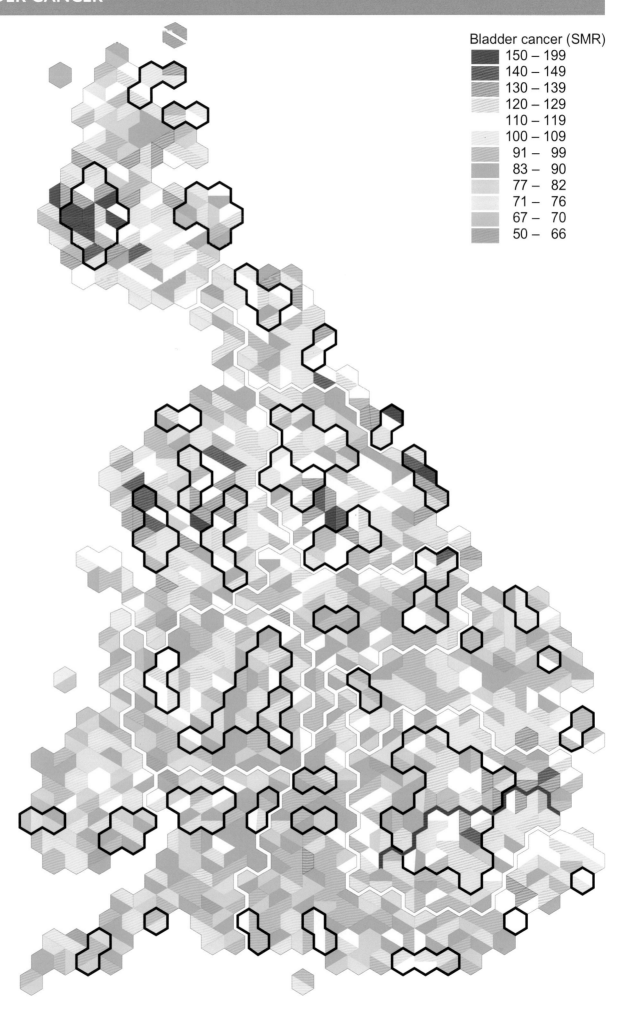

Bladder cancer (SMR)

- 150 – 199
- 140 – 149
- 130 – 139
- 120 – 129
- 110 – 119
- 100 – 109
- 91 – 99
- 83 – 90
- 77 – 82
- 71 – 76
- 67 – 70
- 50 – 66

84 HEART ATTACK AND CHRONIC HEART DISEASE

Heart attack and chronic heart disease are a sub-category of All cardiovascular deaths (See Map 9). 95% of the deaths here are due to atherosclerosis of the coronary arteries.

See also Map 89 Aortic aneurysm and Map 100 Other heart disease.

3,741,101 cases

25.22% of all deaths

average age = 75.3

male:female ratio = 54:46

As a cause of death is more specifically defined, the map of its topography becomes smoother. The neighbourhoods where rates are highest tend to be surrounded by areas with the next highest rates. These are almost all in the north, and rates peak in Scotland, particularly both in and around Glasgow, which is surrounded by a ring of slightly lower rates.

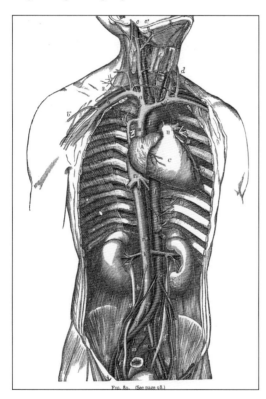

Fig. 80. (See page 98.)

The author Douglas Adams and the educationalist Ted Wragg are among the millions of people to have died of this cause.

Further south, in Wales, Stoke and south Yorkshire are similar rings that highlight the peaks of risk in those areas. Around these areas are found in turn neighbourhoods where rates are average, and next to them areas where you are less likely than most people to die from this most common of causes. Only a few such areas of low risk are found in the north of England, in Scotland and in Wales. Such areas are ubiquitous in the south, where the very lowest rates are found. There are rarely great differences between adjoining areas. Where there are, within the centre of London, is where very rich and very poor live almost side by side.

Heart disease is a major cause of death in Britain and accounts for one quarter of all deaths over the total period studied here. Smoking, high blood pressure, high cholesterol levels, obesity, low physical activity levels and diabetes are important causes of this condition.

Ischaemic heart disease is when there is a build-up of plaques within the walls of the arteries that supply the heart with oxygen and nutrients. People are often not aware that they have the condition until the disease is at an advanced stage; often a sudden heart attack is the first symptom. A heart attack occurs when the blood supply to part of the heart is interrupted, often from complete blockage of an artery by broken-off plaque.

Although a heart attack is often thought to be something that happens to men, almost half of the deaths from this cause are of women (46%), although they tend to die at a slightly older age than do men.

ICD-9 codes: 410-414, 429
ICD-10 codes: I20-I22, I24-I25, I51

ICD-9	ICD-9 name	% of cases	ICD-10	ICD-10 name	% of cases
410	Acute myocardial infarction	59.2	I21	Acute myocardial infarction	44.6
414	Other forms of chronic ischaemic heart disease	36.7	I25.1	Atherosclerotic heart disease	18.4
			I25.9	Chronic ischaemic heart disease, unspecified	32.9
	Other causes in group	4.1		Other causes in group	4.1
		100.0			100.0

MAP 84 HEART ATTACK AND CHRONIC HEART DISEASE

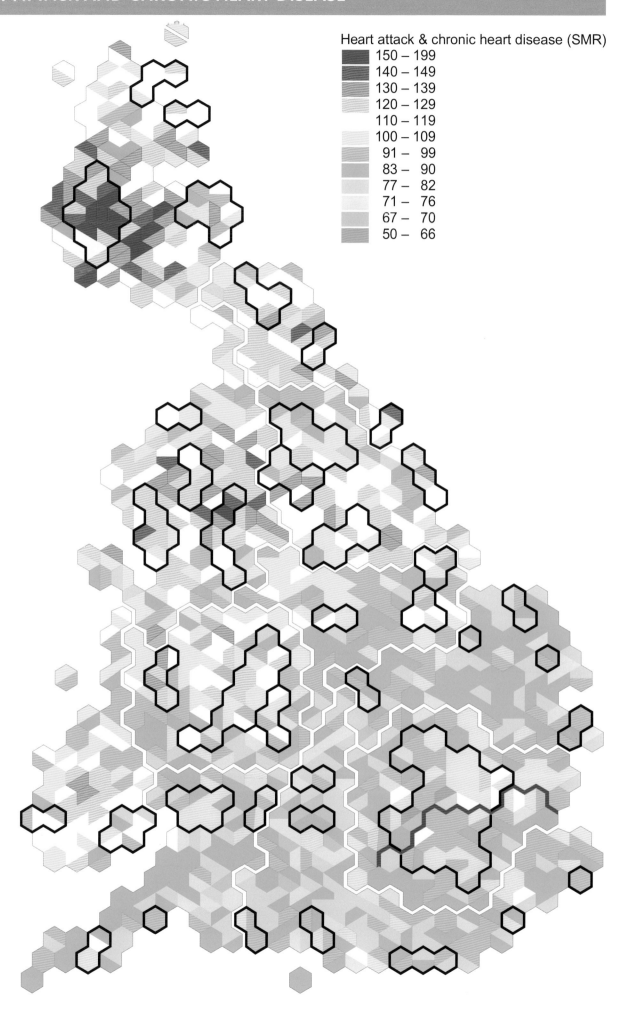

Heart attack & chronic heart disease (SMR)

	150 – 199
	140 – 149
	130 – 139
	120 – 129
	110 – 119
	100 – 109
	91 – 99
	83 – 90
	77 – 82
	71 – 76
	67 – 70
	50 – 66

85 DIABETES MELLITUS

The deaths in this category are due to insulin-dependent diabetes mellitus (also known as Type I diabetes) and non-insulin-dependent diabetes mellitus (also known as Type II diabetes).

See also Map 57 Endocrine disorders (not diabetes).

168,144 cases

1.13% of all deaths

average age = 75.4

male:female ratio = 45:55

Social geographical history plays a key part in the patterning of deaths from diabetes. High rates in north east London, much of the West Midlands, north Manchester and parts of south Wales all point to different geographically concentrated populations who share in common an elevated propensity to die from this cause. Black Caribbean and South Asian people have a higher risk of developing diabetes than White people, and therefore the map reflects, in part, where people from these ethnic groups live. Low rates are found in Aberdeen, Edinburgh, Newcastle, Leeds, Bristol and across the southern chalklands from Somerset to Sussex.

Diabetes mellitus – most commonly referred to as simply diabetes – is a metabolic disorder where the body has abnormally high blood sugar resulting from low levels of the hormone insulin. Type I and II diabetes are chronic conditions. Type I is fatal within months without insulin injections. Type II diabetes can be managed by dietary treatment, tablets and insulin supplementation where necessary. A third type is gestational diabetes, which occurs during pregnancy. This may normalise after delivery but women experiencing gestational diabetes have an increased risk of Type II diabetes in later life.

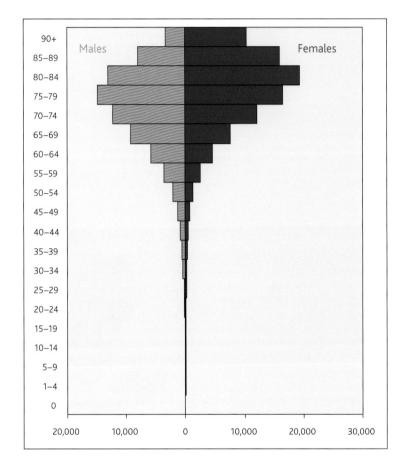

The acute complications of diabetes include ketoacidosis (when there is very high blood sugar due to insulin deficiency) and hypoglycaemia (when blood sugar is too low due to treatment). Both can lead to coma. Chronic complications include increased risk of cardiovascular disease, chronic renal failure, damage to the retina which in turn leads to blindness, and nerve damage, particularly of the feet. Peripheral vascular disease can cause gangrene and may require amputation.

Many people who have Type II diabetes are unaware that they have the condition.

ICD-9 codes: 250
ICD-10 codes: E10-E11, E13-E14

ICD-9	ICD-9 name	% of cases	ICD-10	ICD-10 name	% of cases
250	Diabetes mellitus	100.0	E10	Insulin-dependent diabetes mellitus	7.9
			E11	Non-insulin-dependent diabetes mellitus	20.0
			E14	Unspecified diabetes mellitus	72.0
				Other causes in group	0.1
		100.0			100.0

MAP 85   DIABETES MELLITUS

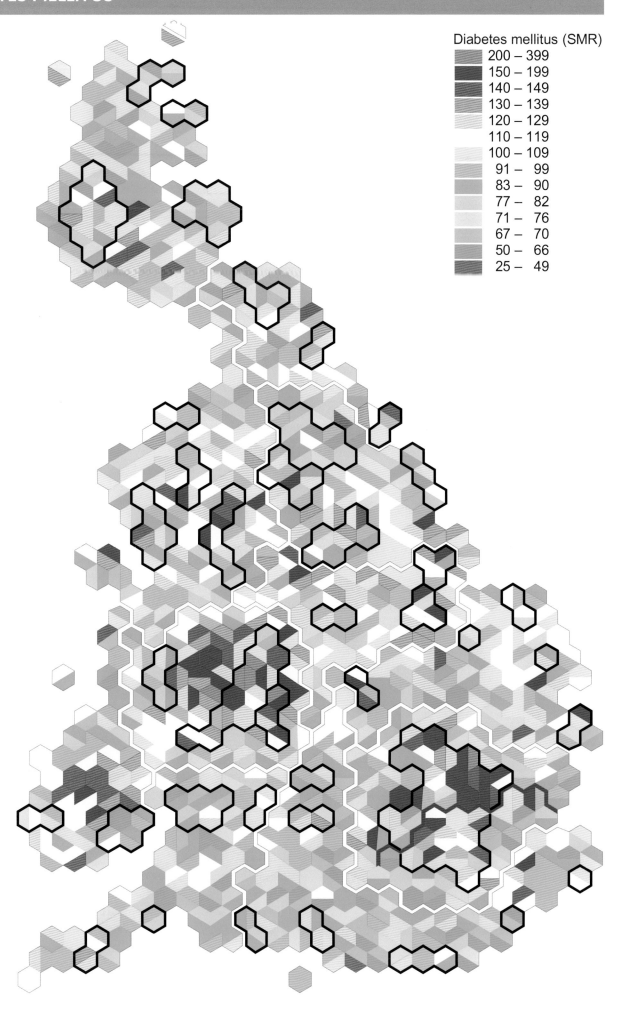

Diabetes mellitus (SMR)
- 200 – 399
- 150 – 199
- 140 – 149
- 130 – 139
- 120 – 129
- 110 – 119
- 100 – 109
- 91 – 99
- 83 – 90
- 77 – 82
- 71 – 76
- 67 – 70
- 50 – 66
- 25 – 49

86   HYPERTENSIVE DISEASE

Hypertensive disease is when the blood pressure is chronically elevated.

It is a sub-category of All cardiovascular deaths (Map 9).

94,721 cases

0.64% of all deaths

average age = 75.7

male:female ratio = 44:56

There is a patterning to deaths from this disease that does not fit the standard. North London, the Black Country, south Wales, south Cambridgeshire, central Manchester and Glasgow do not have a huge amount in common other than having high rates of death from this disease. Similarly, those areas where death from this illness are rarer have little in common other than that the pace of life tends to perhaps be slower, Swindon being the town where hypertensive disease is most rarely the cause of death. Local idiosyncrasies in diagnosis and cause of death certification may have a part to play, and so may idiosyncrasies in treatment or lack thereof. Black African and Black Caribbean people have a higher risk of high blood pressure. Lifestyle factors are also important. High blood pressure is often asymptomatic and therefore not diagnosed or treated.

Hypertension, or high blood pressure, can be the result of other underlying (that is, secondary) health problems, such as kidney disease. Obesity is an important cause of high blood pressure.

High blood pressure means the heart has to work harder to pump blood around the body, which can weaken it. Hypertension often causes no immediate problems but is an important risk factor for strokes, heart attacks, heart failure, arterial aneurysm and chronic renal failure. The main risk factors are obesity, alcohol, a high salt diet and a family history of high blood pressure.

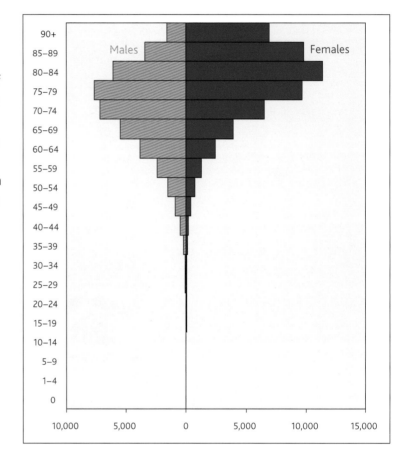

High blood pressure is usually detected through routine health check ups. Treatment can be through long-term medication but lifestyle changes are also recommended: weight reduction, reducing salt in the diet and reducing alcohol consumption all help. Exercise and not smoking reduce the associated risks.

ICD-9 codes: 401-404
ICD-10 codes: I10-I13

ICD-9	ICD-9 name	% of cases	ICD-10	ICD-10 name	% of cases
401	Essential hypertension	9.4	I10	Essential (primary) hypertension	13.9
402	Hypertensive heart disease	73.0	I11	Hypertensive heart disease	65.5
403	Hypertensive renal disease	12.8	I12	Hypertensive renal disease	15.3
			I13	Hypertensive heart and renal disease	5.3
	Other causes in group	4.8			
		100.0			100.0

MAP 86A (FEMALES) 86B (MALES)   HYPERTENSIVE DISEASE

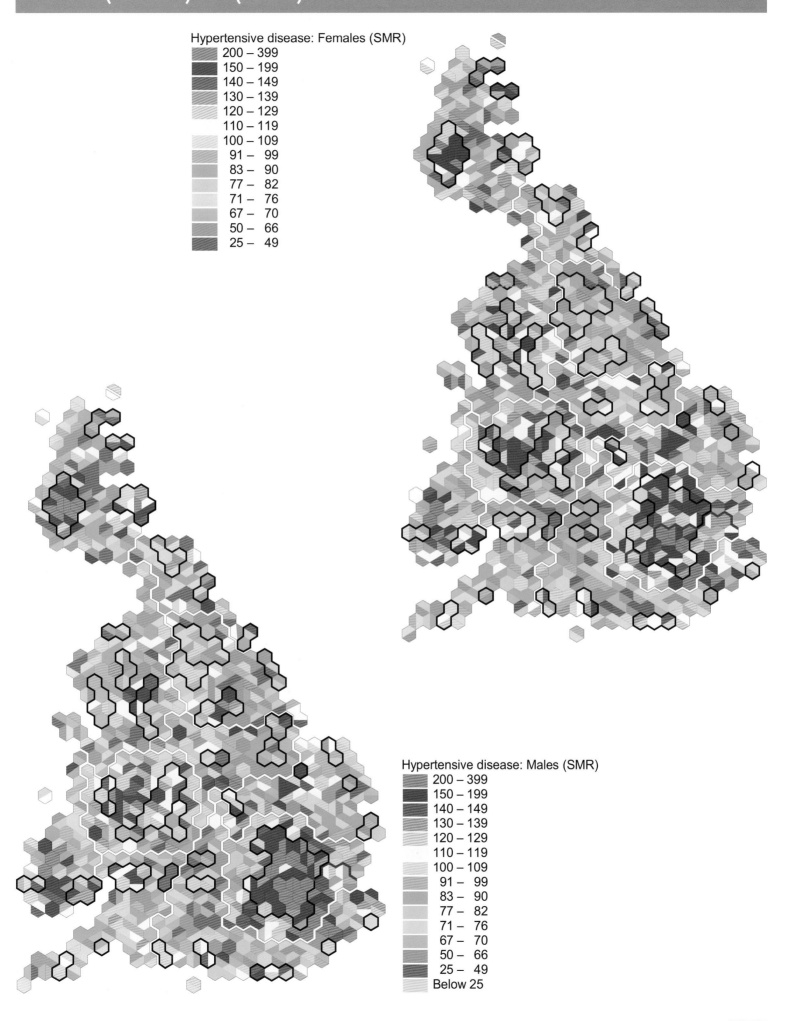

Hypertensive disease: Females (SMR)
- 200 – 399
- 150 – 199
- 140 – 149
- 130 – 139
- 120 – 129
- 110 – 119
- 100 – 109
- 91 – 99
- 83 – 90
- 77 – 82
- 71 – 76
- 67 – 70
- 50 – 66
- 25 – 49

Hypertensive disease: Males (SMR)
- 200 – 399
- 150 – 199
- 140 – 149
- 130 – 139
- 120 – 129
- 110 – 119
- 100 – 109
- 91 – 99
- 83 – 90
- 77 – 82
- 71 – 76
- 67 – 70
- 50 – 66
- 25 – 49
- Below 25

87   DISEASES OF BLOOD

This category includes a range of disorders which affect the blood.

See also Map 58 Leukaemia.

48,759 cases

0.33% of all deaths

average age = 76.0

male:female ratio = 42:58

Deaths from this cause are a little less common in the more affluent parts of the south and a little more common in some parts of some of Britain's larger cities. However, average rates are found up and down the country.

One of the diseases included here is sickle cell anaemia, which is considerably more common in those of Black African and Black Caribbean ethnicities, and so if we were to map that alone it would reflect the geography of these ethnic groups in Britain.

Other diseases in this category are more often the end result of some disease rather than diseases in their own right. They include:

- aplastic anaemia: a condition where the bone marrow does not produce sufficient new cells to replenish blood cells;
- disseminated intravascular coagulation: where the blood starts to coagulate throughout the whole body;
- agranulocytosis: a reduction in the number of white blood cells in the body.

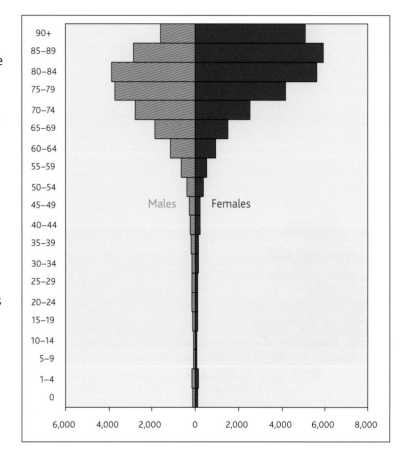

The age–sex bar chart shows that more older women are affected by this cause than are men.

ICD-9 codes: 280-289

ICD-10 codes: D50-D53, D56-D61, D64-D73, D75, D89.2, I88

ICD-9	ICD-9 name	% of cases	ICD-10	ICD-10 name	% of cases
281	Other deficiency anaemias	7.1			
284	Aplastic anaemia	10.2	D61	Other aplastic anaemias	15.2
285	Other and unspecified anaemias	21.4	D64	Other anaemias	30.6
286	Coagulation defects	5.3	D65	Disseminated intravascular coagulation [defibrination syndrome]	5.1
287	Purpura and other haemorrhagic conditions	5.4	D69	Purpura and other haemorrhagic conditions	10.5
289	Other diseases of blood and blood-forming organs	38.3	D70	Agranulocytosis	9.9
	Other causes in group	12.3		Other causes in group	28.7
		100.0			100.0

MAP 87   DISEASES OF BLOOD

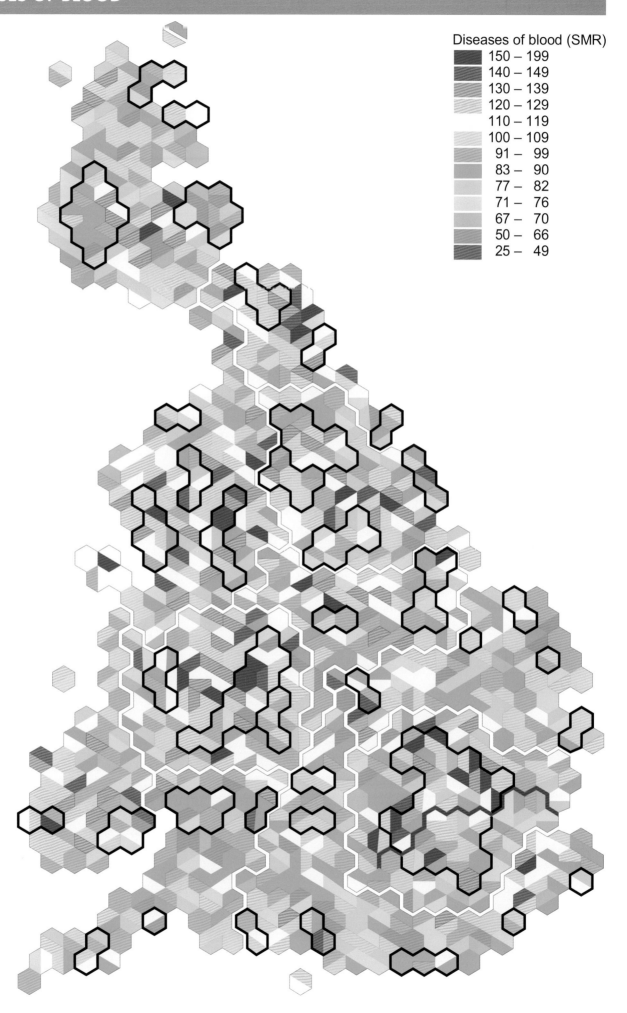

Diseases of blood (SMR)
- 150 – 199
- 140 – 149
- 130 – 139
- 120 – 129
- 110 – 119
- 100 – 109
- 91 – 99
- 83 – 90
- 77 – 82
- 71 – 76
- 67 – 70
- 50 – 66
- 25 – 49

88 CHRONIC LOWER RESPIRATORY DISEASES

This is a sub-category of All respiratory deaths (see Map 10). Most of the diseases are of the lungs.

See also Map 55 Asthma, Map 63 Bronchitis, Map 94 Industrial lung diseases, Map 97 Other respiratory disorders, Map 102 Influenza and Map 105 Pneumonia.

683,198 cases

4.61% of all deaths

average age = 76.0

male:female ratio = 62:38

Most of the deaths in this category are from chronic obstructive pulmonary disease (COPD), of which the leading cause is smoking. The other main cause of such deaths is industrial pollution. Rates are highest in Glasgow, the industrial areas of northern England and the Midlands, south Wales and London. In contrast, rates are very low in most of the south of the country. The geographical pattern of female deaths is slightly more pronounced than that for those of males.

COPD is an umbrella term for a chronic lung disease such as emphysema and chronic bronchitis. It is also known as chronic obstructive airway disease (COAD) or chronic obstructive lung disease (COLD). COPD occurs when the airways are obstructed or have narrowed. The damage caused by COPD is permanent. It is a common disease and affects approximately one million people in the UK. As the age–sex bar chart shows, while the age distributions are a similar shape for men and women, more men succumb to this cause of death than do women.

A lifelong smoker, King Edward VII suffered from severe bronchitis which undoubtedly contributed to his death. Actor Vincent Price, artist Norman Rockwell, actor Robert Mitchum, poet T.S. Eliot, novelist Fyodor Dostoevsky, singer Dean Martin and actor Arthur English all died from emphysema.

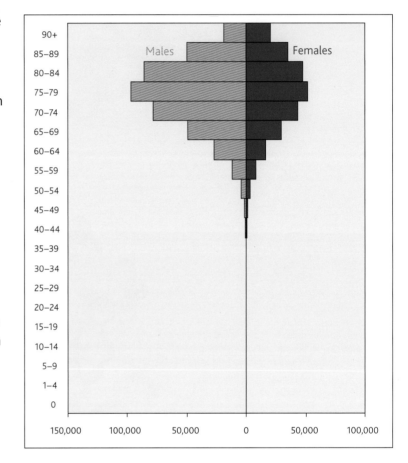

ICD-9 codes: 490-492, 494, 496
ICD-10 codes: J40-J44, J47

ICD-9	ICD-9 name	% of cases	ICD-10	ICD-10 name	% of cases
491	Chronic bronchitis	24.1			
492	Emphysema	7.0	J43	Emphysema	5.4
496	Chronic airways obstruction, not elsewhere classified	65.1	J44.9	Chronic obstructive pulmonary disease, unspecified	82.0
	Other causes in group	3.8		Other causes in group	12.6
		100.0			100.0

MAP 88A (FEMALES) 88B (MALES) CHRONIC LOWER RESPIRATORY DISEASES

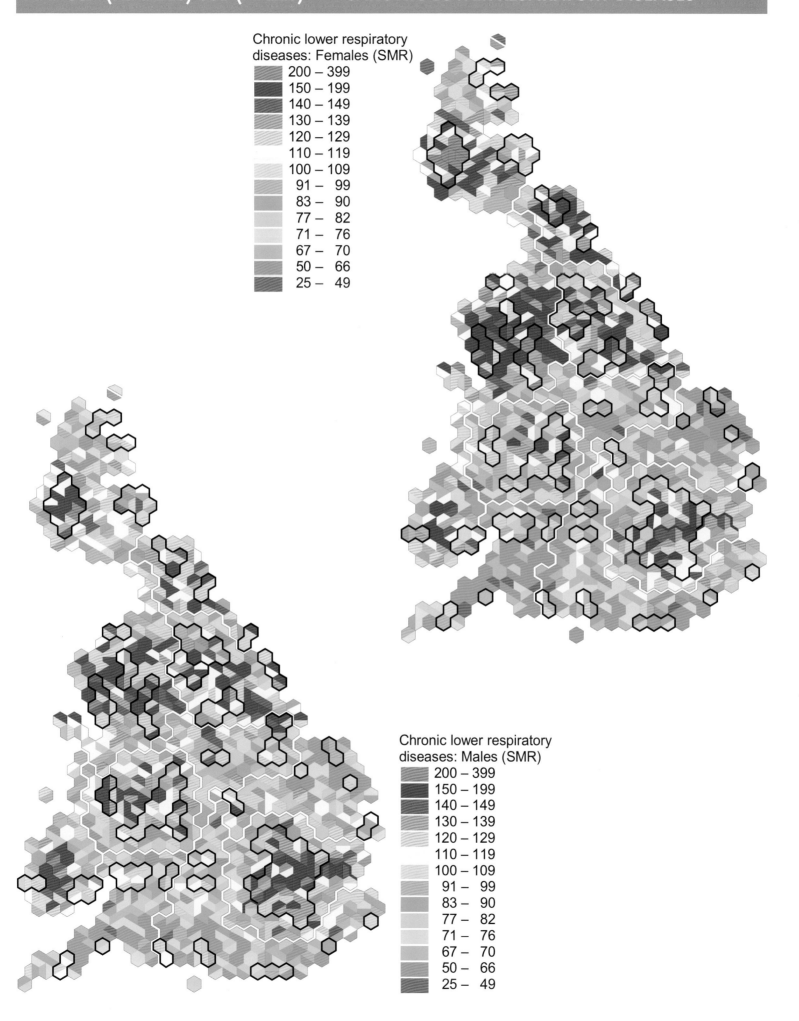

Chronic lower respiratory
diseases: Females (SMR)

	200 – 399
	150 – 199
	140 – 149
	130 – 139
	120 – 129
	110 – 119
	100 – 109
	91 – 99
	83 – 90
	77 – 82
	71 – 76
	67 – 70
	50 – 66
	25 – 49

Chronic lower respiratory
diseases: Males (SMR)

	200 – 399
	150 – 199
	140 – 149
	130 – 139
	120 – 129
	110 – 119
	100 – 109
	91 – 99
	83 – 90
	77 – 82
	71 – 76
	67 – 70
	50 – 66
	25 – 49

89 AORTIC ANEURYSM

Aortic aneurysm is a term that refers to any swelling of the aorta. Where this swelling is sufficient to have led to death this is recorded as the underlying cause.

See also Map 84 Heart attack and chronic heart disease, Map 98 Cerebrovascular disease and Map 108 Atherosclerosis.

215,370 cases

1.45% of all deaths

average age = 76.1

male:female ratio = 63:37

Here there is a geographical gradient opposite to that seen in most of these pages. Rates are lowest in Scotland, rise as you move south, and peak in Kent. In between there are clusters of slight differences to what is otherwise a remarkably smooth pattern.

The aorta is the largest artery in the heart, originating in the left ventricle, going into the chest and then into the abdominal cavity. An aneurysm, or balloon-like bulge, can occur anywhere along the aorta. The swelling caused by aortic aneurysm may cause this blood vessel to rupture, resulting in severe pain, and a quick death.

The age–sex bar chart shows that this is a condition very rarely affecting people below the age of 60, and with more males than females being susceptible to this cause of death.

Aortic aneurysm is treated with surgery, preferably before the aorta actually ruptures. Controlling blood pressure and cholesterol, and not smoking, reduce the risk. However, given the apparent similarity of risk factors for aortic aneurysm and coronary heart disease it is striking that this map and the map of all cardiovascular deaths (Map 9) are so different.

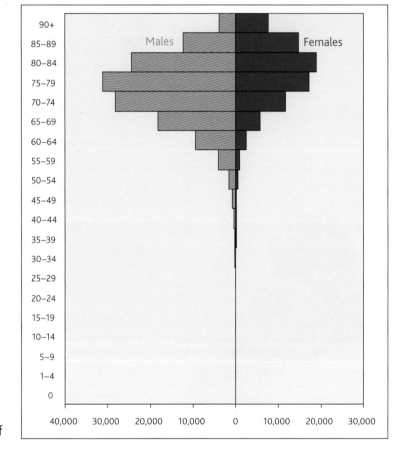

ICD-9 codes: 441
ICD-10 codes: I71

ICD-9	ICD-9 name	% of cases	ICD-10	ICD-10 name	% of cases
441	Aortic aneurysm	100.0	I71	Aortic aneurysm and dissection	100.0
		100.0			100.0

MAP 89A (FEMALES) 89B (MALES)   AORTIC ANEURYSM

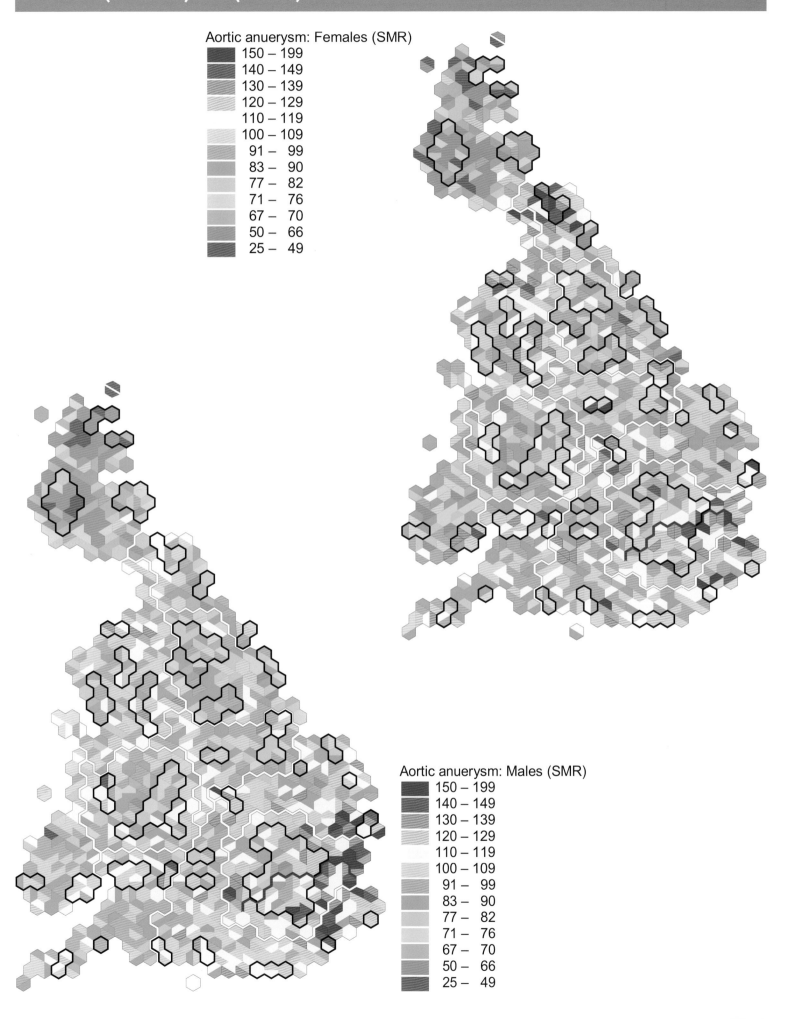

Aortic anuerysm: Females (SMR)

■	150 – 199
■	140 – 149
▨	130 – 139
▨	120 – 129
	110 – 119
	100 – 109
	91 – 99
	83 – 90
	77 – 82
	71 – 76
	67 – 70
	50 – 66
■	25 – 49

Aortic anuerysm: Males (SMR)

■	150 – 199
■	140 – 149
▨	130 – 139
▨	120 – 129
	110 – 119
	100 – 109
	91 – 99
	83 – 90
	77 – 82
	71 – 76
	67 – 70
	50 – 66
■	25 – 49

90   OTHER DIGESTIVE DISORDERS

This category includes a range of disorders affecting the digestive system.

See also Map 72 Pancreatic cancer, Map 74 Rectal cancer and Map 78 Stomach cancer.

> 315,624 cases
>
> 2.13% of all deaths
>
> average age = 76.8
>
> male:female ratio = 38:62

The highest rates are found in and around Glasgow, with further clusters in the Manchester area. High rates are also found in the neighbourhoods of Nottingham New Basford, Birkenhead North-East and Liverpool Riverside North. The lowest rates are found in an arc stretching from north Wales, through the Marches and the south west of England across to the Home Counties.

The diseases in this category include diseases of the teeth and mouth, the oesophagus, stomach and duodenum, appendix, intestines, peritoneum, liver, gall bladder and pancreas.

The age–sex bar chart shows that younger people rarely die from these digestive disorders. Rates increase with age and are higher for older women aged 75 or above than for older men.

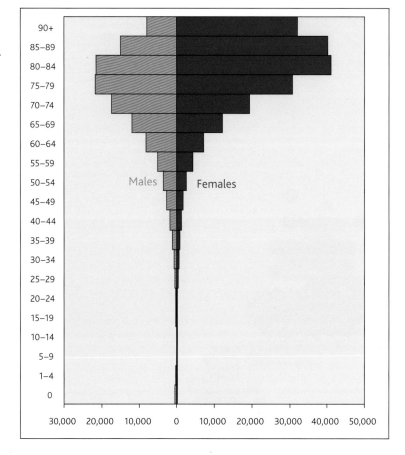

ICD-9 codes: 520-530, 535-537, 540-543, 550-553, 555-558, 560, 562, 564-570, 572-579

ICD-10 codes: K00, K04-K05, K07-K08, K10-K12, K14, K20-K22, K29-K31, K35, K37-K38, K40-K46, K50-K52, K55-K63, K65-K66, K71-K72, K75, K76.1, K76.3-K76.9, K80-K83, K85-K86, K90, K92

ICD-9	ICD-9 name	% of cases	ICD-10	ICD-10 name	% of cases
557	Vascular insufficiency of intestine	13.7	K55.0	Acute vascular disorders of intestine	5.6
			K55.9	Vascular disorder of intestine, unspecified	7.0
560	Intestinal obstruction without mention of hernia	10.5	K56	Paralytic ileus and intestinal obstruction without hernia	11.1
562	Diverticula of intestine	12.9	K57	Diverticular disease of intestine	12.0
569	Other disorders of intestine	5.3	K63	Other diseases of intestine	6.5
577	Diseases of pancreas	7.9	K85	Acute pancreatitis	6.3
578	Gastro-intestinal haemorrhage	10.2	K92.2	Gastro-intestinal haemorrhage, unspecified	10.2
	Other causes in group	39.5		Other causes in group	41.3
		100.0			100.0

MAP 90 OTHER DIGESTIVE DISORDERS

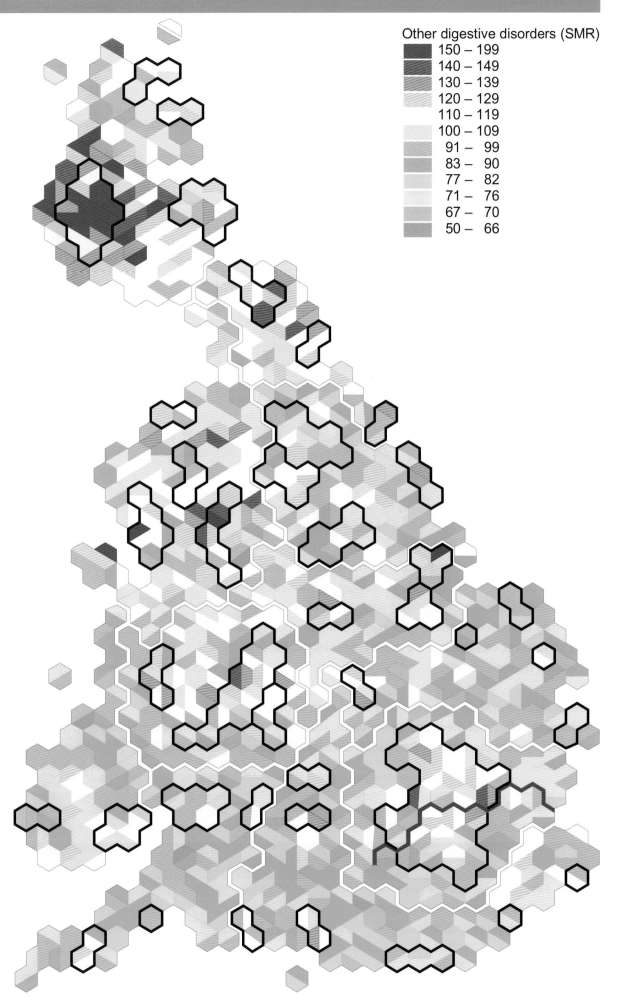

Other digestive disorders (SMR)
- 150 – 199
- 140 – 149
- 130 – 139
- 120 – 129
- 110 – 119
- 100 – 109
- 91 – 99
- 83 – 90
- 77 – 82
- 71 – 76
- 67 – 70
- 50 – 66

92 OTHER CIRCULATORY DISORDERS

This category includes circulatory disorders not included elsewhere.

See also Map 75 Rheumatic heart disease, Map 82 Pulmonary circulatory disorders, Map 84 Heart attack and chronic heart disease, Map 86 Hypertensive disease, Map 89 Aortic aneurysm, Map 98 Cerebrovascular disease, Map 100 Other heart disease and Map 108 Atherosclerosis.

250,956 cases

1.69% of all deaths

average age = 76.8

male:female ratio = 42:58

Other circulatory disorders tend to be a more common cause of death in urban areas. For females the highest rates are found in Ormskirk and Skelmersdale in Lancashire, central Manchester, Inner London south of the Thames and Medway in Kent. The remainder of Britain has average or below average rates. The urban–rural divide is stronger on the male map, with Glasgow having the highest rates, followed by west London, Nottingham and Manchester.

Although this is a residual category of 'All cardiovascular deaths' it nonetheless accounts for over a quarter of a million deaths over the 24-year time period studied here. In the most recent period a third of all deaths in this group were from phlebitis – inflammation of a vein, usually in the legs – and thrombophlebitis – a bloodclot in a vein.

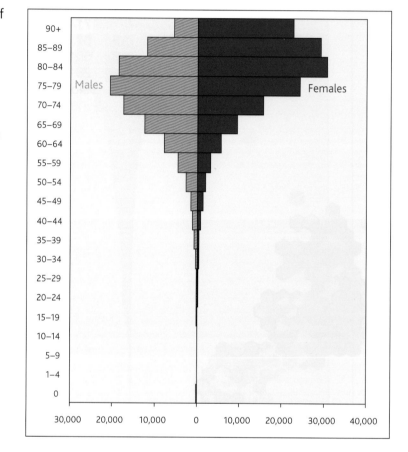

ICD-9 codes: 424, 442-444, 446-448, 451-459

ICD-10 codes: I34-I38, I72-I74, I77-I78, I80-I87, I89, I95, I99, M30-M31, R58

ICD-9	ICD-9 name	% of cases	ICD-10	ICD-10 name	% of cases
424	Other diseases of endocardium	32.5	I35	Nonrheumatic aortic valve disorders	22.8
443	Other peripheral vascular disease	25.2	I73	Other peripheral vascular diseases	23.6
451	Phlebitis and thrombophlebitis	14.1	I80	Phlebitis and thrombophlebitis	33.8
453	Other venous embolism and thrombosis	12.4			
	Other causes in group	15.8		Other causes in group	19.8
		100.0			100.0

MAP 92A (FEMALES) 92B (MALES)   OTHER CIRCULATORY DISORDERS

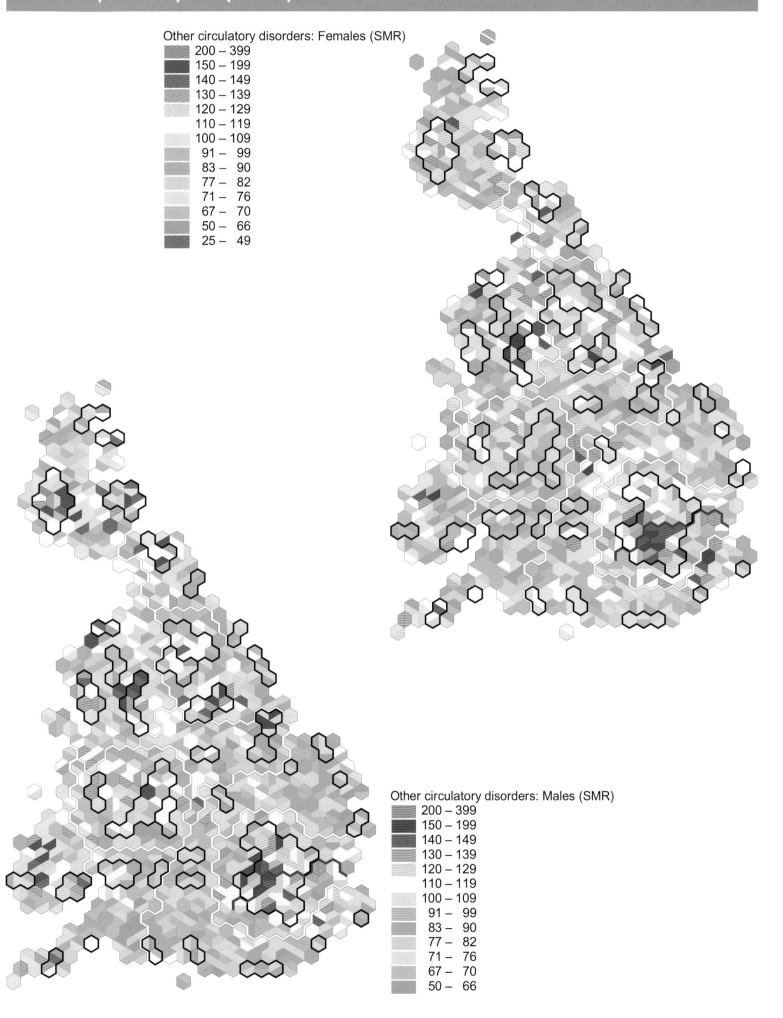

Other circulatory disorders: Females (SMR)

- 200 – 399
- 150 – 199
- 140 – 149
- 130 – 139
- 120 – 129
- 110 – 119
- 100 – 109
- 91 – 99
- 83 – 90
- 77 – 82
- 71 – 76
- 67 – 70
- 50 – 66
- 25 – 49

Other circulatory disorders: Males (SMR)

- 200 – 399
- 150 – 199
- 140 – 149
- 130 – 139
- 120 – 129
- 110 – 119
- 100 – 109
- 91 – 99
- 83 – 90
- 77 – 82
- 71 – 76
- 67 – 70
- 50 – 66

93 STOMACH ULCERS

These are peptic ulcers which occur in the upper gastrointestinal tract, where the mucous membrane has broken down. They can lead to haemorrhage and death.

See also Map 78 Stomach cancer.

108,517 cases

0.73% of all deaths

average age = 77.0

male:female ratio = 46:54

The highest rates on the male map are found in Glasgow, the north west of England, Nottingham, Inner London, Stoke and Newcastle. More rural areas tend to have lower rates. The female map does not have the high rates of males, although Glasgow, Manchester, and Nottingham all have higher rates than average, while in London the prevalence is lower than for males and more dispersed.

Peptic ulcers all occur in places where stomach acid can get. They occur in the oesophagus, stomach (gastric ulcers), duodenum and occasionally the jejunum. These lesions can cause pain, bleed and perforate (sometimes totally). Aspirin and alcohol can exacerbate them. Many of these types of ulcer are associated with the *Helicobacter pylori* bacterium which lives in the acidic environment of the stomach and is generally acquired in infancy or childhood.

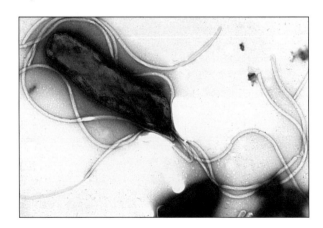

Helicobacter pylori

The actor Rudolph Valentino and the author J. R. R. Tolkien died from ulcers.

ICD-9 codes: 531-534
ICD-10 codes: K25-K28

ICD-9	ICD-9 name	% of cases	ICD-10	ICD-10 name	% of cases
531	Gastric ulcer	32.6	K25	Gastric ulcer	27.3
532	Duodenal ulcer	51.4	K26	Duodenal ulcer	57.4
533	Peptic ulcer, site unspecified	15.5	K27	Peptic ulcer, site unspecified	14.8
	Other causes in group	0.5		Other causes in group	0.5
		100.0			100.0

MAP 93A (FEMALES) 93B (MALES)   STOMACH ULCERS

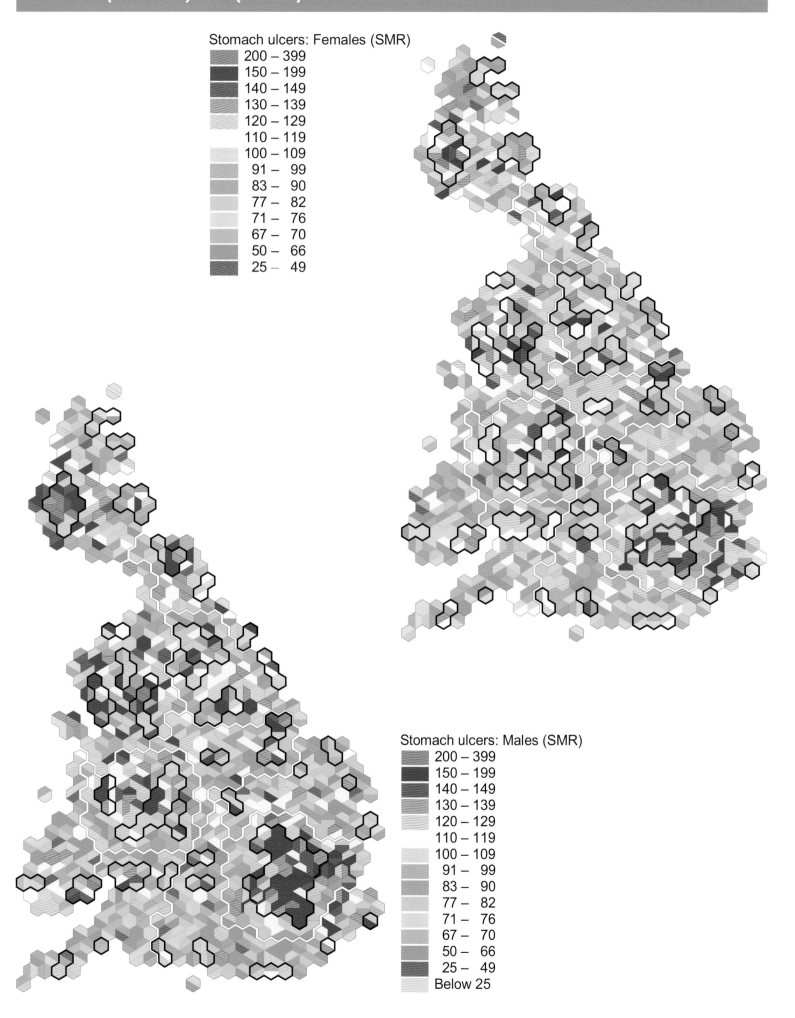

Stomach ulcers: Females (SMR)
- 200 – 399
- 150 – 199
- 140 – 149
- 130 – 139
- 120 – 129
- 110 – 119
- 100 – 109
- 91 – 99
- 83 – 90
- 77 – 82
- 71 – 76
- 67 – 70
- 50 – 66
- 25 – 49

Stomach ulcers: Males (SMR)
- 200 – 399
- 150 – 199
- 140 – 149
- 130 – 139
- 120 – 129
- 110 – 119
- 100 – 109
- 91 – 99
- 83 – 90
- 77 – 82
- 71 – 76
- 67 – 70
- 50 – 66
- 25 – 49
- Below 25

94   INDUSTRIAL LUNG DISEASES

The category of industrial lung diseases includes diseases of the lung due to the inhalation of dust (such as coal dust) or chemicals, which damage the lungs.

See also Map 10 All respiratory deaths and Map 68 Lung cancer.

24,352 cases

0.16% of all deaths

average age = 77.0

male:female ratio = 68:32

To a large extent this is a map of the industrial history of Britain. The male and female maps are very different, due to the differing industrial exposure of the two sexes. Male rates are highest in the coal-mining areas of the south Wales valleys, Yorkshire, Durham and the central belt of Scotland. Stoke also has high rates, probably related to the pottery industry, as does the Sunderland area, likely a legacy of the shipbuilding industry. The southern part of the country generally has very low rates. Female rates tend not to be as high as male rates, and are more dispersed. The highest female rates are found in the north west around Manchester, reflecting mill work, and in Glasgow.

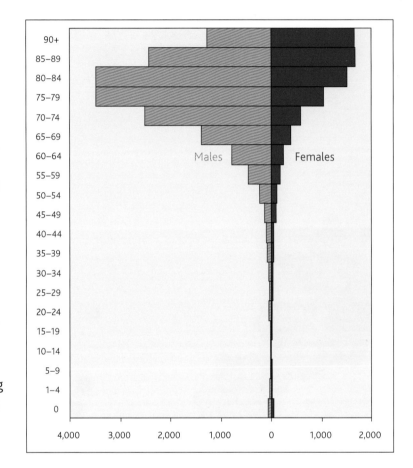

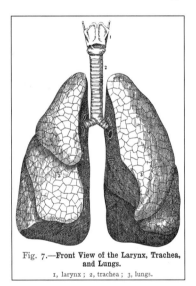

Fig. 7.—Front View of the Larynx, Trachea, and Lungs.

1, larynx ; 2, trachea ; 3, lungs.

While the coal-mining industry is perhaps the most notorious cause of industrial lung disease, a range of other industrial settings can also be hazardous in this respect, such as working with spraying paints onto textiles, exposure to chemical batteries and popcorn factory work.

ICD-9 codes: 500-508

ICD-10 codes: J60-J66, J68-J70

ICD-9	ICD-9 name	% of cases	ICD-10	ICD-10 name	% of cases
500	Coalworkers' pneumoconiosis	30.5	J60	Coalworker's pneumoconiosis	7.8
501	Asbestosis	7.9			
505	Pneumoconiosis, unspecified	6.0			
507	Pneumonitis due to solids and liquids	49.1	J69	Pneumonitis due to solids and liquids	85.3
	Other causes in group	6.5		Other causes in group	6.9
		100.0			100.0

MAP 94A (FEMALES) 94B (MALES)   INDUSTRIAL LUNG DISEASES

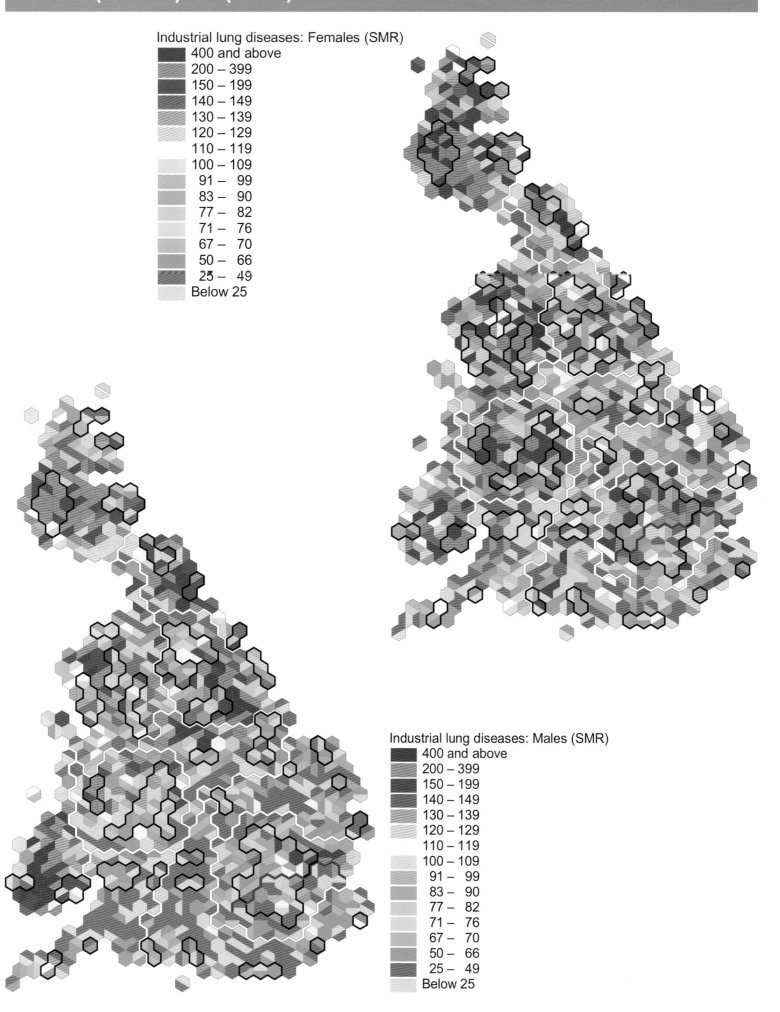

Industrial lung diseases: Females (SMR)
- 400 and above
- 200 – 399
- 150 – 199
- 140 – 149
- 130 – 139
- 120 – 129
- 110 – 119
- 100 – 109
- 91 – 99
- 83 – 90
- 77 – 82
- 71 – 76
- 67 – 70
- 50 – 66
- 25 – 49
- Below 25

Industrial lung diseases: Males (SMR)
- 400 and above
- 200 – 399
- 150 – 199
- 140 – 149
- 130 – 139
- 120 – 129
- 110 – 119
- 100 – 109
- 91 – 99
- 83 – 90
- 77 – 82
- 71 – 76
- 67 – 70
- 50 – 66
- 25 – 49
- Below 25

95   PROSTATE CANCER

This cause is cancer of the prostate gland, which is part of the male reproductive system. Abnormal growths in the prostate leading to death are all included here.

See also Map 7 All cancer deaths.

203,975 cases

1.38% of all deaths

average age = 77.1

male:female ratio = 100:0

There is only slight geographical variation in death rates from prostate cancer. The southern half of Britain tends to have higher rates and the northern half lower. Men of Black ethnicities are more likely to develop prostate cancer than are White men, while Asian men are less likely to do so.

Prostate cancer results from the abnormal growth of cells within the prostate. It is a slow-growing cancer and may remain undiagnosed for a long period of time; many men die with prostate cancer rather than from it. Often this form of cancer does not cause any symptoms or problems, particularly in the early stages, but in some cases it does grow quickly and move to other parts of the body.

There are various treatments available for prostate cancer. Active monitoring involves regular check-ups but no actual treatment until the cancer is found to be growing. Treatment options for more advanced disease include surgery, radiotherapy, brachytherapy (a form of radiotherapy where a radioactive source, such as a small seed, is placed inside or next to the area requiring treatment) and hormone therapy.

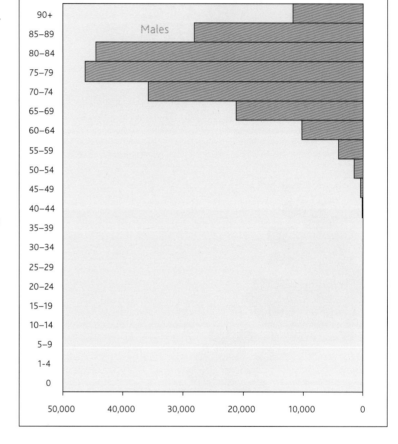

Black activist Stokely Carmichael, comedian Bob Monkhouse and musician Frank Zappa died of prostate cancer.

ICD-9 codes: 185
ICD-10 codes: C61

ICD-9	ICD-9 name	% of cases	ICD-10	ICD-10 name	% of cases
185	Malignant neoplasm of prostate	100.0	C61	Malignant neoplasm of prostate	100.0
		100.0			100.0

MAP 95   PROSTATE CANCER

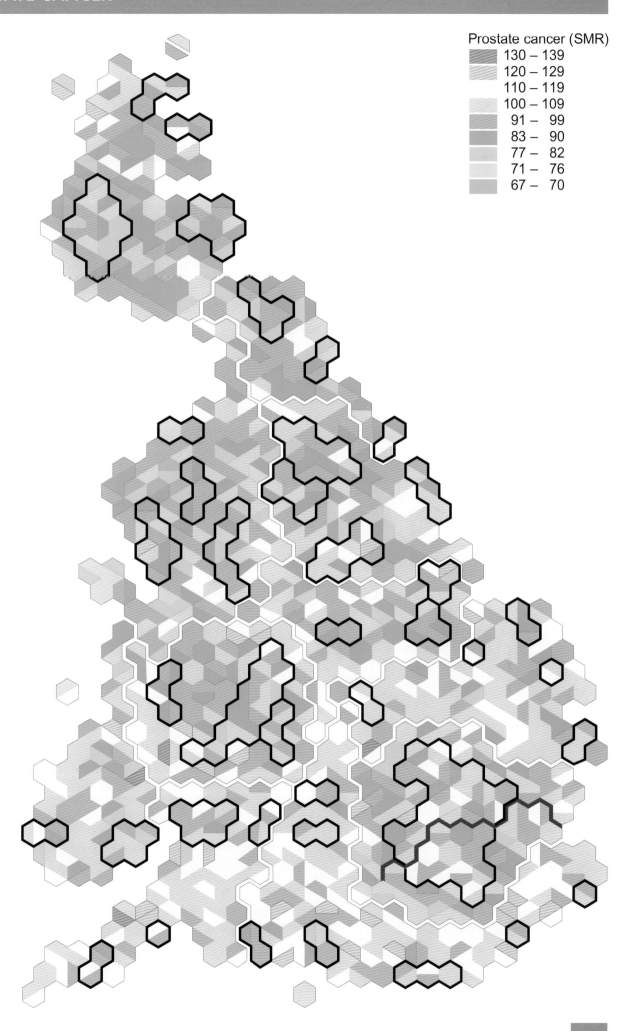

Prostate cancer (SMR)
- 130 – 139
- 120 – 129
- 110 – 119
- 100 – 109
- 91 – 99
- 83 – 90
- 77 – 82
- 71 – 76
- 67 – 70

96   DISEASES OF KIDNEY AND URETER

This category includes different types of renal (kidney) failure as well as diseases of the ureter, which connects the kidneys to the bladder.

See also Map 83 Bladder cancer, Map 85 Diabetes mellitus and Map 103 Other genitourinary disorders.

131,623 cases

0.89% of all deaths

average age = 78.1

male:female ratio = 44:56

The high mortality rate across the majority of Scotland for this cause of death is the most striking feature of the distribution of these diseases in Britain. This is made all the more stark by average or low rates across almost all of Edinburgh, and very low rates in former industrial cities such as Sheffield and Bristol. Although mortality rates from these causes are generally lower in more affluent places, there are stronger geographical factors that influence mortality and susceptibility to these various diseases than any simple relation to wealth and poverty.

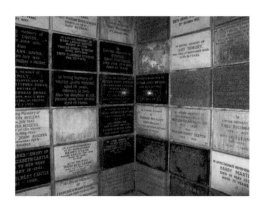

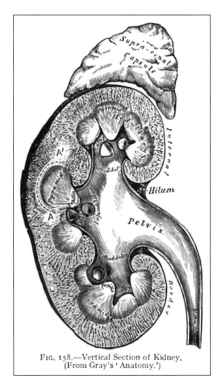

FIG. 158.—Vertical Section of Kidney.
(From Gray's 'Anatomy.')

There are various causes of chronic renal failure, including diabetes, high blood pressure, infection, blockage (such as that caused by kidney stones) and polycystic kidney disease. Depending on the cause, it can be treated by medication and lifestyle changes, by dialysis, or kidney transplant.

Kidney disease is more common in people of South Asian, African and Afro-Caribbean origin.

The actress Sarah Bernhardt and the Soviet leader Yuri Andropov died of kidney disease.

ICD-9 codes: 580-594

ICD-10 codes: N00-N01, N03-N05, N07, N10-N12, N13.0-N13.8, N14-N15, N17-N21, N25-N28, N39.1

ICD-9	ICD-9 name	% of cases	ICD-10	ICD-10 name	% of cases
584	Acute renal failure	10.1	N17	Acute renal failure	13.4
585	Chronic renal failure	33.0	N18	Chronic renal failure	39.1
586	Renal failure, unspecified	29.0	N19	Unspecified renal failure	26.4
590	Infections of kidney	13.5			
	Other causes in group	14.4		Other causes in group	21.1
		100.0			100.0

MAP 96 DISEASES OF KIDNEY AND URETER

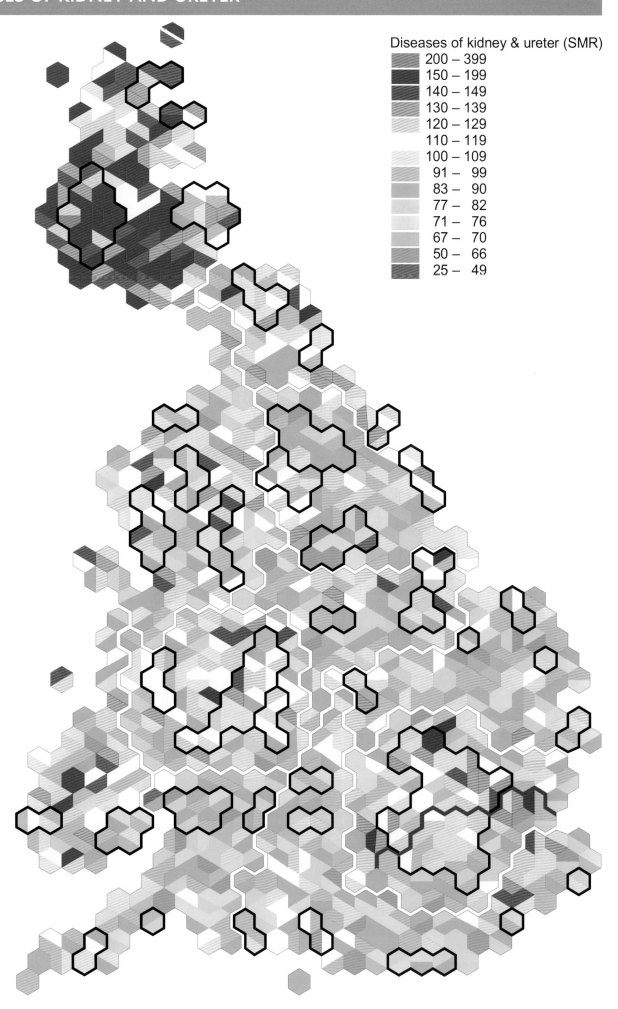

Diseases of kidney & ureter (SMR)
- 200 – 399
- 150 – 199
- 140 – 149
- 130 – 139
- 120 – 129
- 110 – 119
- 100 – 109
- 91 – 99
- 83 – 90
- 77 – 82
- 71 – 76
- 67 – 70
- 50 – 66
- 25 – 49

98 CEREBROVASCULAR DISEASE

This category includes deaths from stroke and other diseases relating to problems affecting the blood vessels that supply the brain.

See also Map 84 Heart attack and chronic heart disease, Map 89 Aortic aneurysm and Map 108 Atherosclerosis.

1,703,628 cases

11.48% of all deaths

average age = 79.2

male:female ratio = 38:62

With the odd geographical exception, as you travel south and east from the west coast of Scotland down to the Sussex beaches, rates of death from this cause fall. The odd exceptions include the more affluent suburbs of Newcastle and similarly favoured places in Yorkshire; conversely some of the less economically favoured spots within Bradford, Manchester, Bolton, Birmingham and Nottingham have higher rates than the surrounding areas. This map reveals threefold variations in mortality rates from the disease across a very smoothly changing national gradient.

This category accounts for more than 10% of all deaths, with 62% of those being of females.

A 'stroke' occurs when there is a loss of brain function due to a disturbance in the supply of blood to the brain. It can result in a range of problems such as difficulty walking, balance problems, speech problems and confusion. Risk factors for stroke include high blood pressure, diabetes, smoking, heavy alcohol consumption and obesity.

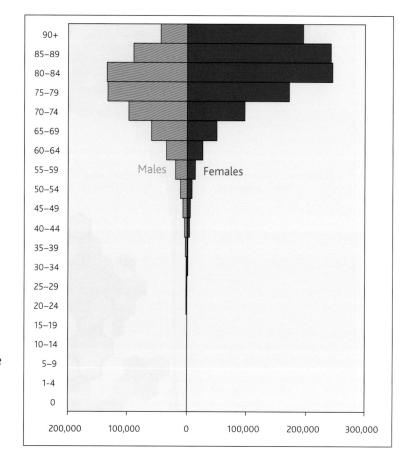

ICD-9 codes: 430-438

ICD-10 codes: G45, I60-I64, I66, I67.0-I67.2, I67.4-I67.5, I67.7-I67.9, I69

ICD-9	ICD-9 name	% of cases	ICD-10	ICD-10 name	% of cases
431	Intracerebral haemorrhage	8.0	I61	Intracerebral haemorrhage	7.8
434	Occlusion of cerebral arteries	13.4	I63.9	Cerebral infarction, unspecified	8.5
436	Acute but ill-defined cerebrovascular disease	59.9	I64	Stroke, not specified as haemorrhage or infarction	54.2
437.9	Other and ill-defined cerebrovascular disease – Unspecified	7.1	I67.9	Cerebrovascular disease, unspecified	15.3
			I69	Sequelae of cerebrovascular disease	5.7
	Other causes in group	11.6		Other causes in group	8.5
		100.0			100.0

MAP 98   CEREBROVASCULAR DISEASE

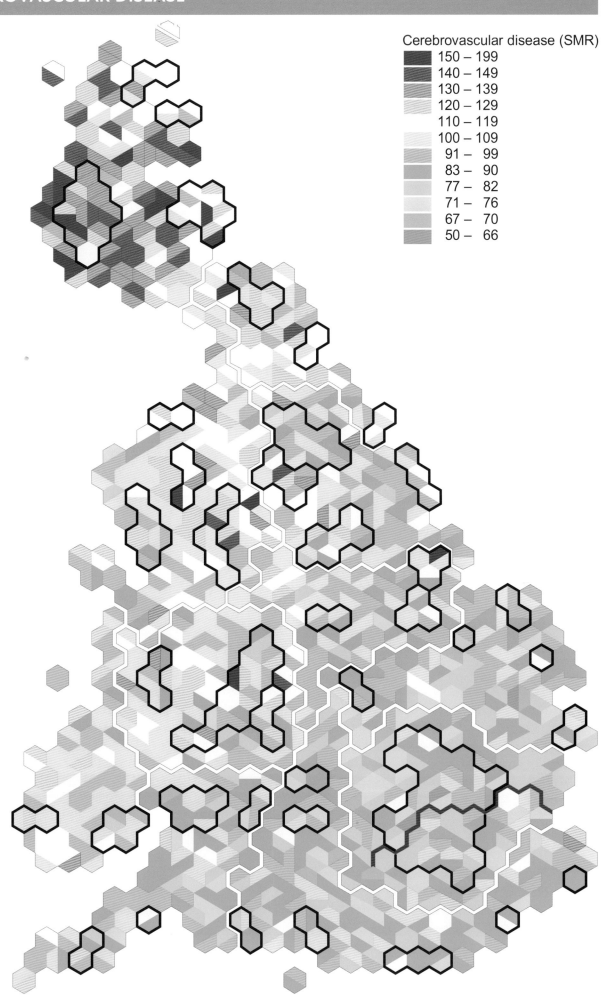

Cerebrovascular disease (SMR)
- 150 – 199
- 140 – 149
- 130 – 139
- 120 – 129
- 110 – 119
- 100 – 109
- 91 – 99
- 83 – 90
- 77 – 82
- 71 – 76
- 67 – 70
- 50 – 66

99 OTHER TISSUE, SKIN, MUSCULOSKELETAL DISORDERS

This category includes rheumatism, skin ulcers and bone disorders such as osteoporosis. The largest sub-category in this group is, itself, a grouping of other causes and so a quite disparate set of underlying causes all related to similar organs are included here.

134,724 cases

0.91% of all deaths

average age = 79.7

male:female ratio = 25:75

Sheffield and Southend stand out clearly with the highest rates, with Bristol not far behind. If we compare this map to Map 91, of falls, we can see that these places have low SMRs for that cause. In contrast, rates in Scotland, Wales and around much of the coasts are especially low. The group of diseases in this category is very heterogeneous, however, which may account for the unclear picture.

This is a residual category that includes a large number of causes of death. Rheumatoid and osteo-arthritis, osteoporosis, ankylosing spondylitis and scoliosis are painful progressive diseases that limit mobility. Diseases of the skin and connective tissue include cellulitis, skin ulcers, abscesses and psoriasis. These disorders are diseases that kill in old age: females account for three quarters of deaths from this category.

It is likely that the change from ICD-9 to ICD-10 will have caused fewer deaths to be classified as due to falls. We can only speculate that the high rates here are where, with a death following a fall, more doctors in these places have entered osteoporosis, rheumatoid arthritis or osteoarthritis in part I of the death certificate rather than part II.

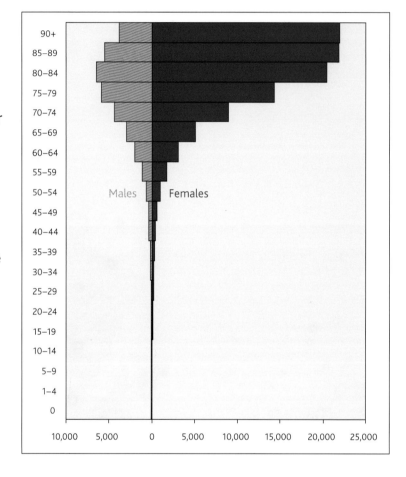

ICD-9 codes: 680-686, 690-698, 700-701, 703, 705-711, 714-733, 735-738

ICD-10 codes: L00-L05, L08, L10, L12-L13, L21, L26-L27, L30, L40, L43, L50-L51, L53, L56-L57, L60, L71-L73, L88-L90, L92-L95, L97-L98, M00, M05-M06, M08, M11-M13, M15-M17, M19-M21, M24-M25, M32-M35, M40-M43, M45-M48, M50-M51, M53-M54, M60-M62, M66-M67, M70-M72, M75-M77, M79-M81, M84-M89, M91-M92, M94-M95

ICD-9	ICD-9 name	% of cases	ICD-10	ICD-10 name	% of cases
			L03.9	Cellulitis, unspecified	5.4
707	Chronic ulcer of skin	10.4	L97	Ulcer of lower limb, not elsewhere classified	6.9
710	Diffuse diseases of connective tissue	5.4			
714	Rheumatoid arthritis and other inflammatory polyarthropathies	22.7	M06	Other rheumatoid arthritis	14.7
715	Osteo-arthrosis and allied disorders	12.4	M25.9	Joint disorder, unspecified	5.5
733	Other disorders of bone and cartilage	24.5	M80	Osteoporosis with pathological fracture	20.0
			M81	Osteoporosis without pathological fracture	5.1
	Other causes in group	24.6		Other causes in group	42.4
		100.0			100.0

MAP 99 OTHER TISSUE, SKIN, MUSCULOSKELETAL DISORDERS

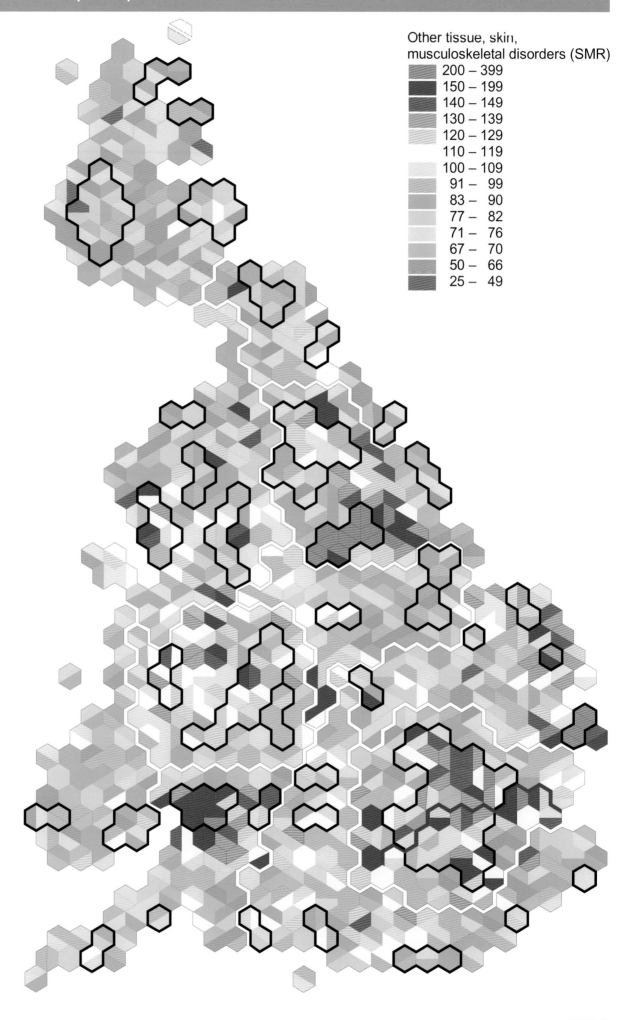

Other tissue, skin,
musculoskeletal disorders (SMR)

■	200 – 399
■	150 – 199
■	140 – 149
■	130 – 139
■	120 – 129
■	110 – 119
■	100 – 109
■	91 – 99
■	83 – 90
■	77 – 82
■	71 – 76
■	67 – 70
■	50 – 66
■	25 – 49

100 OTHER HEART DISEASE

This category includes types of heart disease not included elsewhere; two thirds of deaths in this group are due to heart failure.

See also Map 84 Heart attack and chronic heart disease.

350,146 cases

2.36% of all deaths

average age = 79.7

male:female ratio = 39:61

Five large clusters are clear: urban western Scotland; urban north west England; within the West Midlands conurbation; the western parts of the Welsh valleys; and west Inner London. In contrast eastern Scotland, east of the Pennines, the East Midlands, Bristol (just east of Wales) and the outer south east all record lower than average rates. Other than in these extreme places, that is for most of the country, rates are very close to average and show little geographical variation.

Heart failure refers to the heart not being able to fill with blood or to pump sufficient blood through the body. It can affect the left side of the heart, the right side, or both. Heart failure on the left side can lead to breathlessness. Failure on the right side can cause swollen ankles and legs.

The age–sex bar chart for this cause is very similar to that for the previous three causes mapped, with higher numbers of elderly women succumbing to this form of mortality. This is not surprising as coronary heart disease underlies much heart failure.

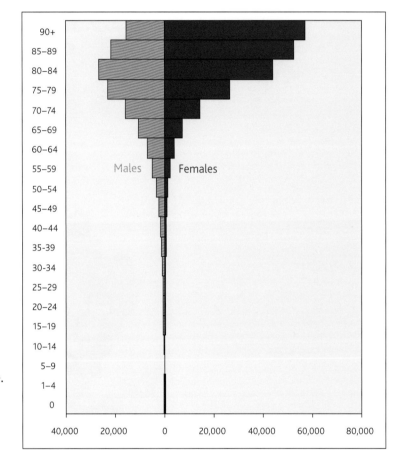

ICD-9 codes: 420-423, 425-428
ICD-10 codes: I30-I31, I33, I40, I42, I44-I50, R00

ICD-9	ICD-9 name	% of cases	ICD-10	ICD-10 name	% of cases
425	Cardiomyopathy	10.3	I42	Cardiomyopathy	9.0
427.3	Atrial fibrillation and flutter	12.8	I48	Atrial fibrillation and flutter	18.8
428	Heart failure	67.8	I50	Heart failure	65.6
	Other causes in group	9.1		Other causes in group	6.6
		100.0			100.0

MAP 100 OTHER HEART DISEASE

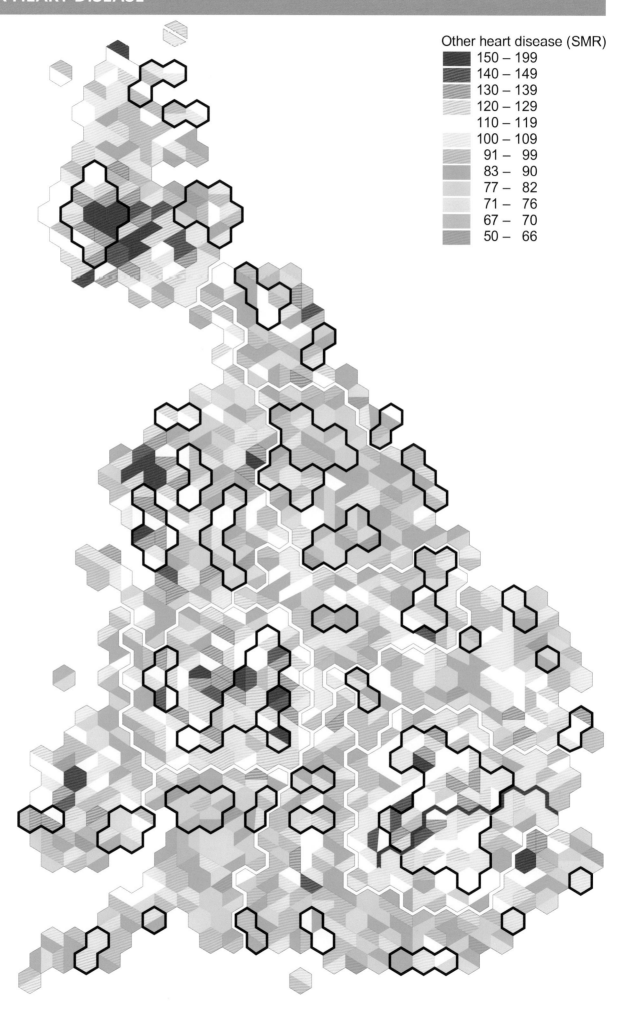

Other heart disease (SMR)

	150 – 199
	140 – 149
	130 – 139
	120 – 129
	110 – 119
	100 – 109
	91 – 99
	83 – 90
	77 – 82
	71 – 76
	67 – 70
	50 – 66

101 PARKINSON'S DISEASE

Parkinson's is a degenerative disease of the brain that affects the nerve cells involved in movement.

See also Map 91 Falls.

84,429 cases

0.57% of all deaths

average age = 80.4

male:female ratio = 54:46

London, Scotland and most towns north and west of Sheffield stand out as being areas with low rates of Parkinson's disease. South Yorkshire, more rural Lancashire, and the Home Counties ring have elevated rates. The map is almost the inverse of that of smoking rates, reflecting the speculation that those more likely to develop Parkinson's disease are a little less likely to take up or sustain the smoking habit.

Parkinson's disease affects a part of the brain that controls certain aspects of movement and so affects walking, talking, writing and swallowing. Symptoms include shaking, slowness of movement and stiffness in the joints. It is a disease that can be difficult to treat.

This cause of death reaps a similar number of men and women; all other causes which follow in this atlas kill more women than men.

Chinese leader Mao Zedong suffered from Parkinson's.

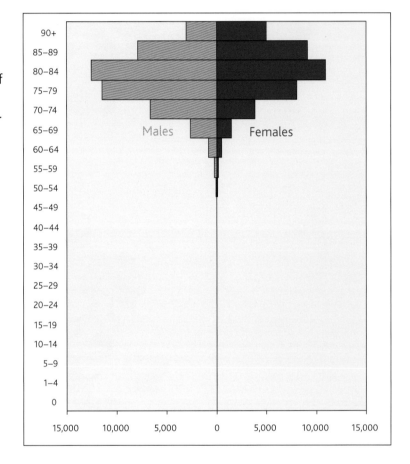

ICD-9 codes: 332
ICD-10 codes: G20, G21.1, G21.3, G21.8-G21.9

ICD-9	ICD-9 name	% of cases	ICD-10	ICD-10 name	% of cases
332	Parkinson's disease	100.0	G20	Parkinson's disease	99.8
				Other causes in group	0.2
		100.0			100.0

MAP 101 PARKINSON'S DISEASE

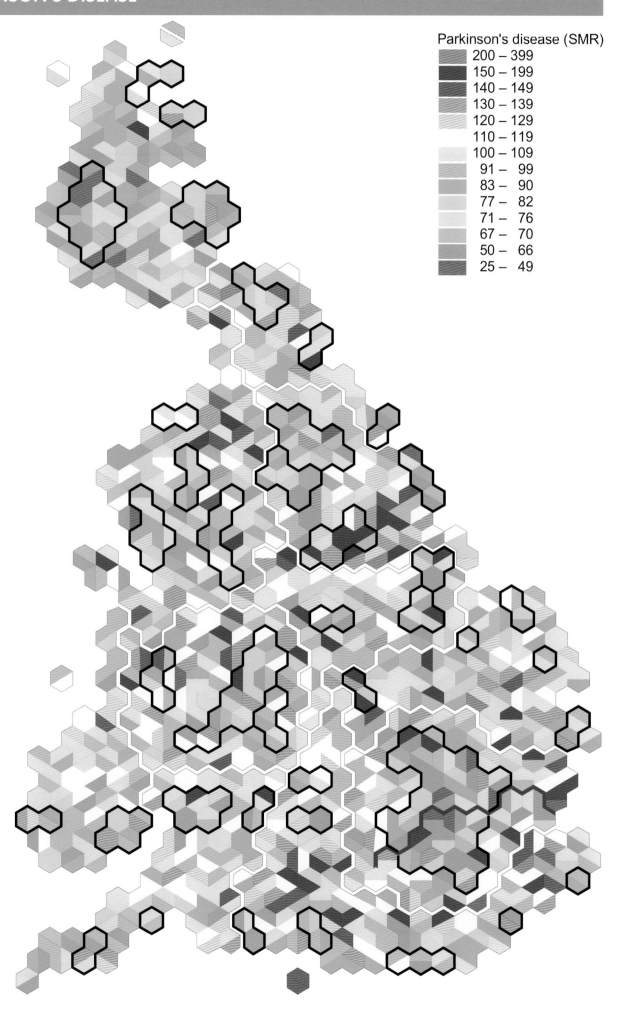

Parkinson's disease (SMR)

	200 – 399
	150 – 199
	140 – 149
	130 – 139
	120 – 129
	110 – 119
	100 – 109
	91 – 99
	83 – 90
	77 – 82
	71 – 76
	67 – 70
	50 – 66
	25 – 49

102 INFLUENZA

Influenza is an infectious disease caused by a virus.

See also Map 105 Pneumonia.

12,140 cases

0.08% of all deaths

average age = 80.7

male:female ratio = 33:67

Here is a map of extremes: in much of the country you are either twice as likely, or half as likely, as the average to meet your death with the assistance of this virus. It is not just in Scotland, particularly its northerly environs, that rates are especially elevated. Little pockets of extremes appear in parts of Norwich and Swindon, Blackpool and even in one of the more salubrious quarters of Oxford.

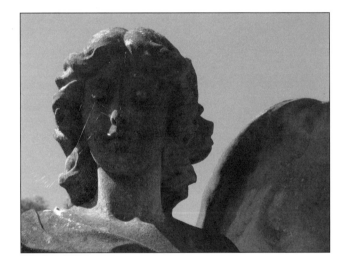

The disease itself being infectious will have tended to have killed in geographical clumps, but those who sign death certificates have a problem. Usually no virus is actually identified, so although influenza may have been present many doctors record the death as due to pneumonia.

The symptoms of influenza are chills, fever, sore throat, muscle pains, headache, coughing and general weakness. It is often confused with the common cold but influenza is much more severe.

Outbreaks of influenza occur in seasonal epidemics; in pandemic years it can kill millions of people. The 1918–19 pandemic is estimated to have claimed 40–50 million lives worldwide. Vaccines are now available but as the virus changes rapidly over time a vaccine that is formulated in one year may be ineffective the next.

ICD-9 codes: 487
ICD-10 codes: J10-J11

ICD-9	ICD-9 name	% of cases	ICD-10	ICD-10 name	% of cases
487	Influenza	100.0	J11	Influenza, virus not identified	95.1
				Other causes in group	4.9
		100.0			100.0

MAP 102 INFLUENZA

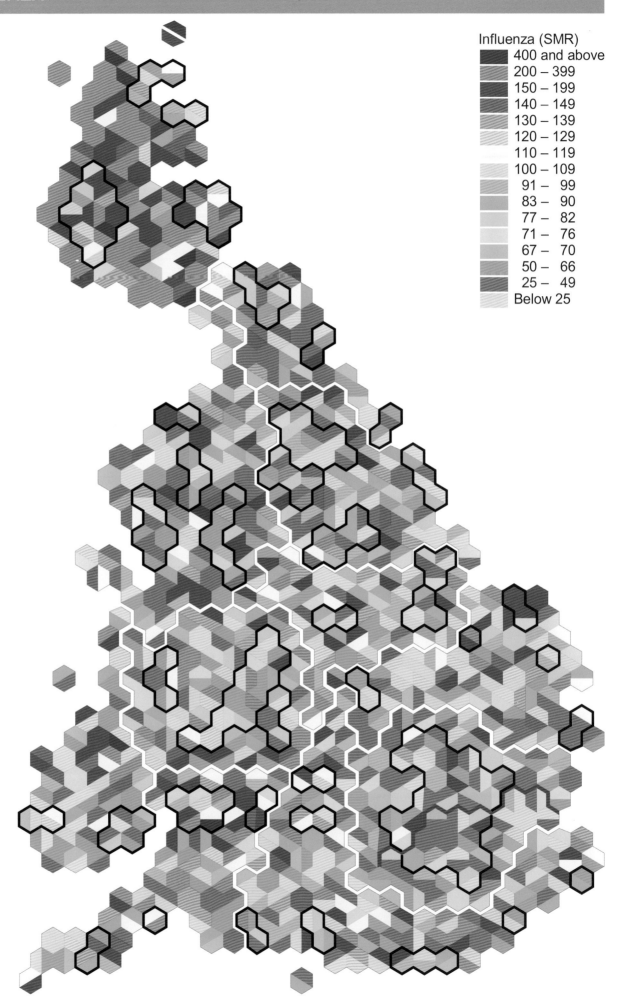

Influenza (SMR)

	400 and above
	200 – 399
	150 – 199
	140 – 149
	130 – 139
	120 – 129
	110 – 119
	100 – 109
	91 – 99
	83 – 90
	77 – 82
	71 – 76
	67 – 70
	50 – 66
	25 – 49
	Below 25

103 OTHER GENITOURINARY DISORDERS

Most of the deaths in this category are due to urinary tract infection, often then leading to kidney failure.

See also Map 83 Bladder cancer, Map 95 Prostate cancer and Map 96 Diseases of kidney and ureter.

72,010 cases

0.49% of all deaths

average age = 81.8

male:female ratio = 45:55

South London, east London and Essex are the blocks of colour on the map opposite that first catch your eye as reflecting unusually large areas of the population suffering elevated rates of mortality from these disorders. At least a dozen other smaller areas can also be singled out for speculation. Just as significant are the places where an unusually large number of people are clustered together who have had a lower than normal chance of dying from these disorders over many years. Such places are more often found around the coasts and away from most city centres.

Urinary tract infection (UTI) is a bacterial infection in the urinary tract that can occur from the urethra through the bladder to the renal pelvis inside the kidney.

Recurrent UTI can lead to kidney stones and kidney failure. UTIs often occur in the hospitalised elderly, for instance after a stroke or a fall.

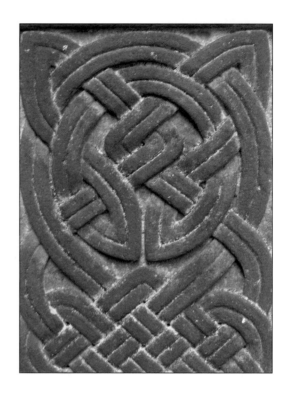

ICD-9 codes: 595-605, 607-608, 611, 614-629

ICD-10 codes: N02, N13.9, N30-N32, N35-N36, N39.0, N39.9, N40-N43, N45, N47-N50, N61, N63-N64, N70-N71, N73, N75-N76, N80-N85, N87-N90, N92-N95, R31

ICD-9	ICD-9 name	% of cases	ICD-10	ICD-10 name	% of cases
599	Other disorders of urethra and urinary tract	69.6	N39.0	Urinary tract infection, site not specified	87.3
600	Hyperplasia of prostate	17.2			
	Other causes in group	13.2		Other causes in group	12.7
		100.0			100.0

MAP 103 OTHER GENITOURINARY DISORDERS

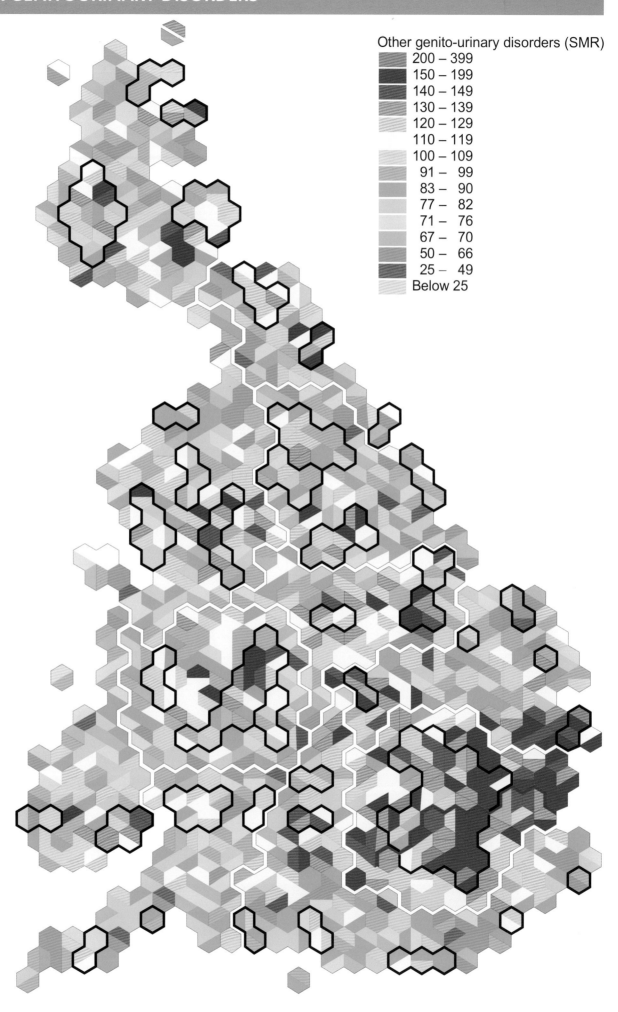

Other genito-urinary disorders (SMR)
- 200 – 399
- 150 – 199
- 140 – 149
- 130 – 139
- 120 – 129
- 110 – 119
- 100 – 109
- 91 – 99
- 83 – 90
- 77 – 82
- 71 – 76
- 67 – 70
- 50 – 66
- 25 – 49
- Below 25

104 OTHER INTESTINAL INFECTIONS

6,623 cases

0.04% of all deaths

average age = 82.3

male:female ratio = 33:67

This group comprises all intestinal infections due to other organisms not included in Map 49. These have been mapped separately from other infections to highlight deaths due to *Clostridium difficile*.

See also Map 6 All deaths due to infections, and Map 49 Deaths due to other infections.

It is partly the rarity of mortality from these causes that leads the map opposite to be so speckled in appearance. High rates concentrate in small clusters, perhaps reflecting outbreaks of food poisoning or contraction from stays in the same hospital: infections are usually local and hence result in localised clustering.

Overall, rates of infection and hence death from infection tend to be lower in more rural and isolated areas. This has been so since time immemorial. Deaths from these diseases used to be more common. Now in many areas they can kill so infrequently that rates are too low to map (that is, with an SMR of below 25).

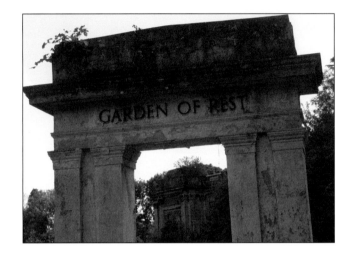

Recently, under ICD-10, enterocolitis due to *Clostridium difficile* has comprised the majority of deaths within this grouping, some 96%. It is not possible to calculate the percentage of deaths from this cause prior to 2000/01, as it was included in the category Other specified bacteria, accounting for four fifths of the deaths in this grouping.

Clostridium difficile is a bacteria that can lead to severe infection of the colon; this often occurs after the flora of the gut have been destroyed by antibiotics. The heat-resistant spores of the organism can survive for long periods of time in settings such as hospitals or nursing homes.

ICD-9 codes: 008
ICD-10 codes: A04, A08

ICD-9	ICD-9 name	% of cases	ICD-10	ICD-10 name	% of cases
008.4	Other specified bacteria	80.0	A04.7	Enterocolitis due to Clostridium difficile	96.1
008.8	Other organism, not elsewhere classified	16.8			
	Other causes in group	3.2		Other causes in group	3.9
		100.0			100.0

MAP 104   OTHER INTESTINAL INFECTIONS

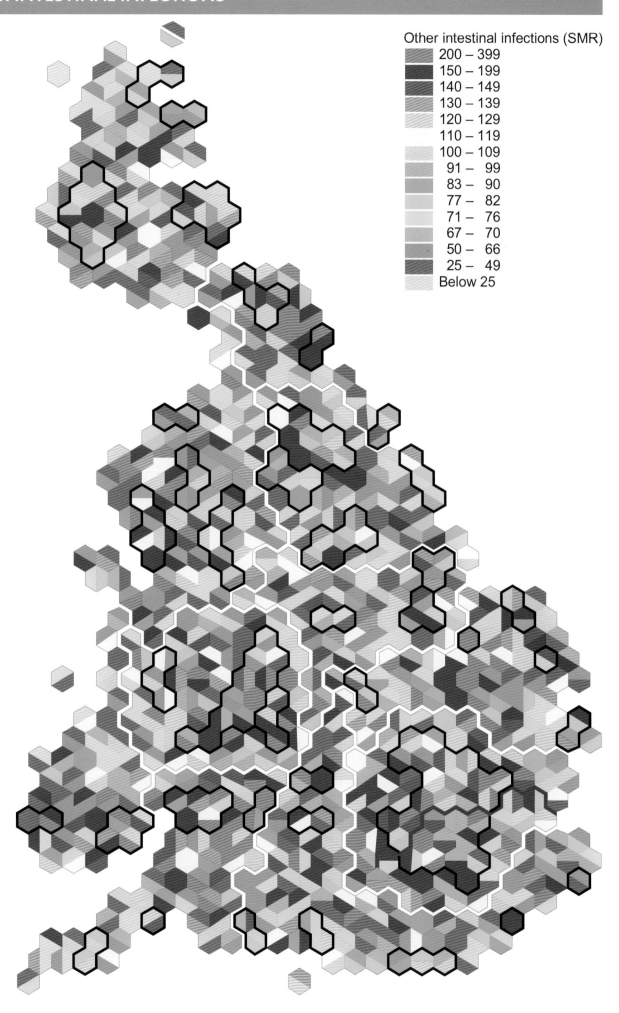

Other intestinal infections (SMR)

	200 – 399
	150 – 199
	140 – 149
	130 – 139
	120 – 129
	110 – 119
	100 – 109
	91 – 99
	83 – 90
	77 – 82
	71 – 76
	67 – 70
	50 – 66
	25 – 49
	Below 25

105 PNEUMONIA

Pneumonia is an inflammatory illness of the lungs. It can occur due to a range of causes including bacteria, viruses, fungi, parasites, exposure to chemicals and injury to the lungs.

See also Map 55 Asthma, Map 63 Bronchitis, Map 88 Chronic lower respiratory diseases, Map 94 Industrial lung disease, Map 97 Other respiratory diseases and Map 102 Influenza.

1,064,320 cases

7.18% of all deaths

average age = 82.6

male:female ratio = 39:61

A little more accurately diagnosed than similar killers, this disease kills mostly those who are poor and have smoked or otherwise suffered damage to their lungs. It can kill at any age, but it tends to reap older people most often. Within the heart of Glasgow, the north of Liverpool, and much of London are found the clearest concentrations of excess mortality from this cause. Rates are especially low in the highlands of Scotland, the south west of England, Norfolk, north Wales, northern Yorkshire and Lancashire.

Pneumonia can usually be treated with antibiotics, but the very young and the frail elderly are particularly vulnerable, as are people with existing illnesses.

Dancer Fred Astaire, television presenter Jeremy Beadle, singer James Brown and writer Leo Tolstoy died from pneumonia.

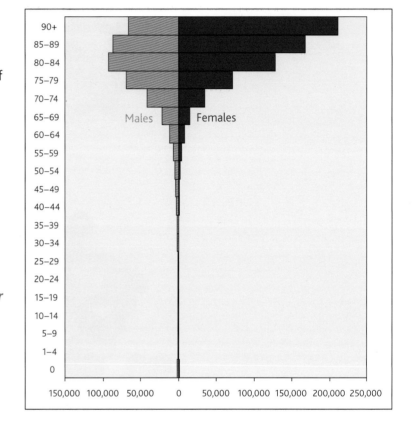

ICD-9 codes: 480-483, 485-486

ICD-10 codes: A48.1-A48.2, J12-J15, J16.8, J18.0-J18.1, J18.8-J18.9

ICD-9	ICD-9 name	% of cases	ICD-10	ICD-10 name	% of cases
481	Pneumococcal pneumonia	5.0	J18.1	Lobar pneumonia, unspecified	6.2
485	Bronchopneumonia, organism unspecified	85.5	J18.0	Bronchopneumonia, unspecified	69.1
486	Pneumonia, organism unspecified	8.7	J18.9	Pneumonia, unspecified	23.6
	Other causes in group	0.8		Other causes in group	1.1
		100.0			100.0

MAP 105A (FEMALES) 105B (MALES)   PNEUMONIA

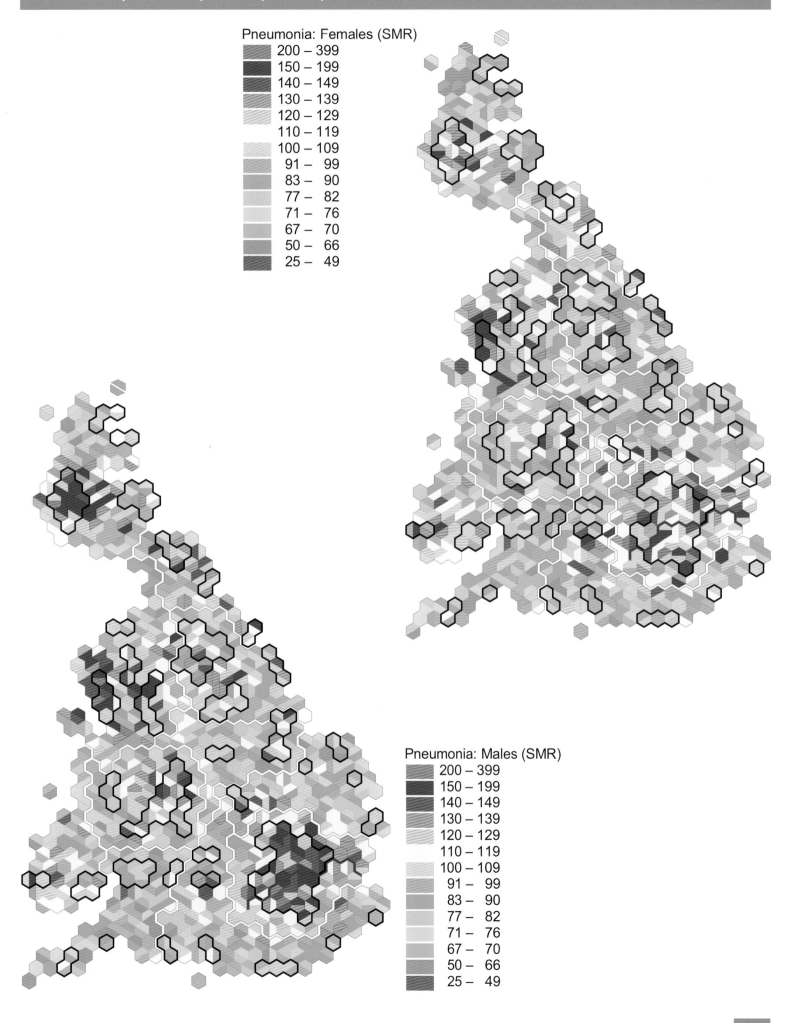

Pneumonia: Females (SMR)

	200 – 399
	150 – 199
	140 – 149
	130 – 139
	120 – 129
	110 – 119
	100 – 109
	91 – 99
	83 – 90
	77 – 82
	71 – 76
	67 – 70
	50 – 66
	25 – 49

Pneumonia: Males (SMR)

	200 – 399
	150 – 199
	140 – 149
	130 – 139
	120 – 129
	110 – 119
	100 – 109
	91 – 99
	83 – 90
	77 – 82
	71 – 76
	67 – 70
	50 – 66
	25 – 49

106 DEMENTIA

Dementia is the loss of intellectual abilities that is severe enough to interfere with social or occupational functioning. Vascular dementia, also called arteriosclerotic or multi infarct dementia, is caused by the poor circulation of blood in the brain.

See also Map 70 Other nervous disorders (which includes Alzheimer's disease) and Map 109 Old age.

161,607 cases

1.09% of all deaths

average age = 84.0

male:female ratio = 30:70

There is no clear pattern to the map here.

Many people with dementia die of pneumonia, and until recently the death was usually classified as due to pneumonia rather than dementia.

While the likelihood of dementia increases with age, it is not a normal part of growing old: most older people never develop dementia.

The dysfunction caused by dementia is multifaceted and involves memory, behaviour, personality, judgement, attention, spatial relations, language and abstract thought. The intellectual decline is usually progressive.

The risk factors for vascular or multi infarct dementia are the same as those for stroke, including high blood pressure, diabetes, smoking, poor diet and excessive alcohol intake.

ICD-9 codes: 290
ICD-10 codes: F01, F05.1

ICD-9	ICD-9 name	% of cases	ICD-10	ICD-10 name	% of cases
290.0	Senile dementia, uncomplicated	77.1	F01	Vascular dementia	99.8
290.1	Presenile dementia	6.8			
290.2	Senile dementia with delusional or depressive features	5.2			
290.4	Arteriosclerotic dementia	10.9			
				Other causes in group	0.2
		100.0			100.0

MAP 106   DEMENTIA

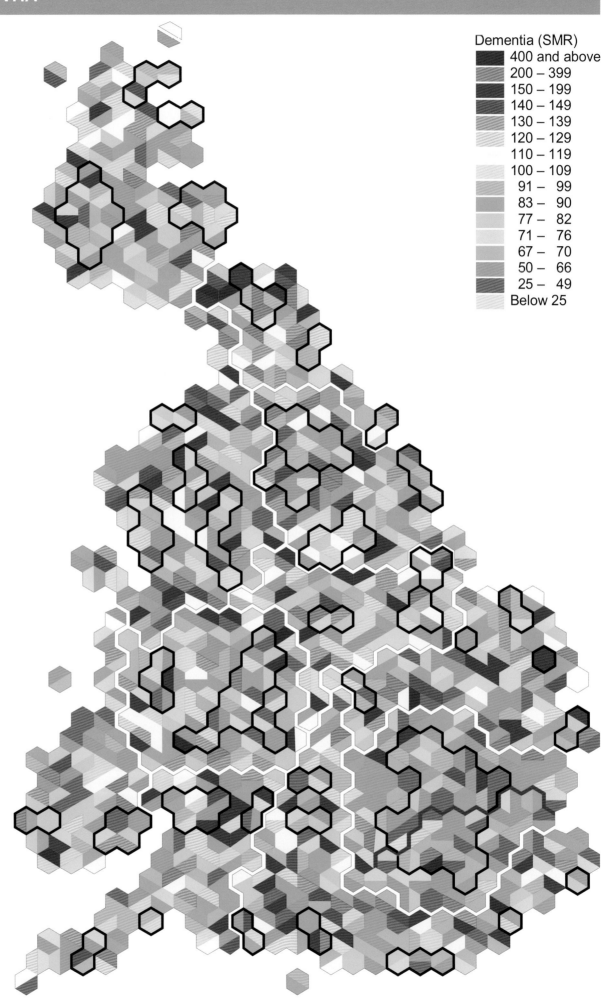

Dementia (SMR)
- 400 and above
- 200 – 399
- 150 – 199
- 140 – 149
- 130 – 139
- 120 – 129
- 110 – 119
- 100 – 109
- 91 – 99
- 83 – 90
- 77 – 82
- 71 – 76
- 67 – 70
- 50 – 66
- 25 – 49
- Below 25

107 OTHER MENTAL DISORDERS

This is a sub-category of All mental disorder deaths (see Map 8) and includes deaths from mental illness.

105,748 cases

0.71% of all deaths

average age = 84.0

male:female ratio = 30:70

In Scotland and in Newcastle these disorders either occur more frequently, kill more people, are diagnosed or are suspected more often, or a combination of all these explanations play their part. Conversely mental disorder is rarely mentioned on the death certificates of those who end their days in and near Brighton, along the north bank of the Thames within London, in west and central Wales, or in Cheshire. At the ages at which these disorders are identified many other afflictions often affect those who die. The extent to which one or the other is more likely to be cited on a death certificate will reflect the medical cultural geography of each area as well as more direct biological mechanisms with environmental influences.

This category includes psychoses, delirium, depressive disorders not elsewhere classified, mental retardation, unspecified dementia and schizophrenia. These disorders reap mostly older people, with nearly 90% of deaths being of those aged 75 and over; 70% of those dying from this cause are females.

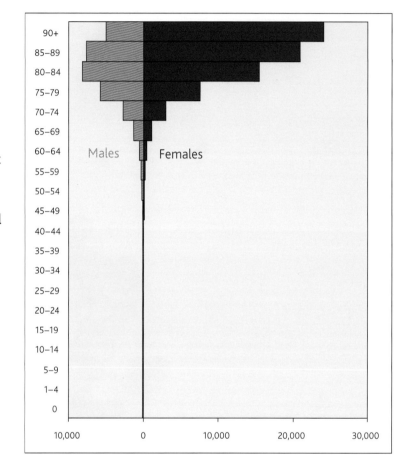

ICD-9 codes: 292-302, 306-312, 314-315, 317-319

ICD-10 codes: F03, F05.9, F06-F07, F09, F11.9, F15.5, F15.9, F17.7, F17.9, F19.3, F19.9, F20, F22-F23, F25, F29-F34, F39, F41-F45, F48, F50, F54, F60, F71-F73, F79, F81, F83, F84.0, F89, F91, F99, R41.0

ICD-9	ICD-9 name	% of cases	ICD-10	ICD-10 name	% of cases
			F03	Unspecified dementia	97.4
295	Schizophrenic psychoses	5.0			
298	Other nonorganic psychoses	74.1			
311	Depressive disorder, not elsewhere classified	8.1			
	Other causes in group	12.8		Other causes in group	2.6
		100.0			100.0

MAP 107 OTHER MENTAL DISORDERS

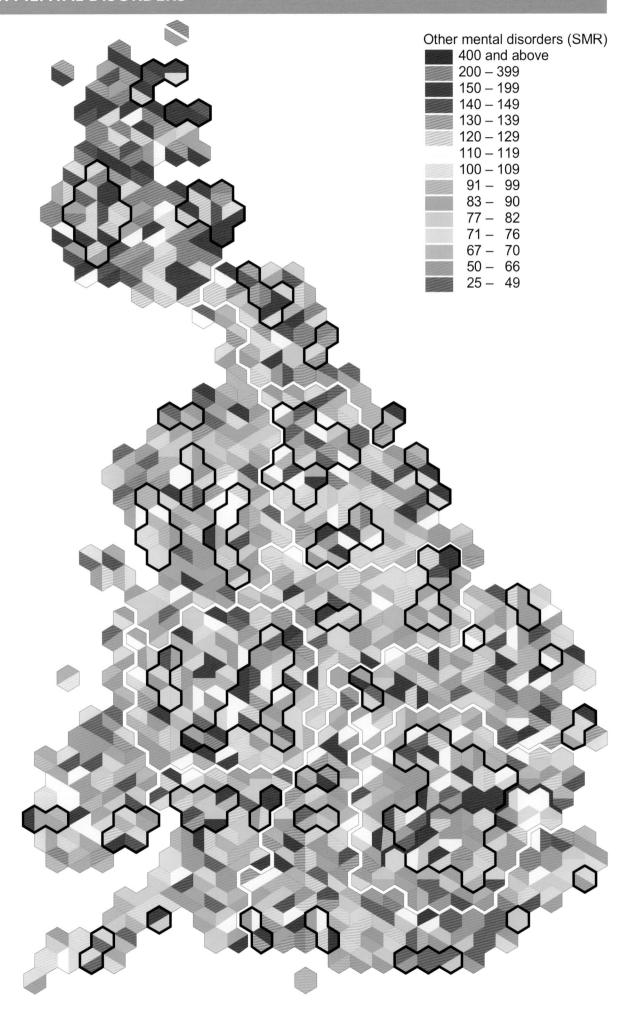

Other mental disorders (SMR)

■	400 and above
	200 – 399
	150 – 199
	140 – 149
	130 – 139
	120 – 129
	110 – 119
	100 – 109
	91 – 99
	83 – 90
	77 – 82
	71 – 76
	67 – 70
	50 – 66
	25 – 49

108 ATHEROSCLEROSIS

93,478 cases

0.63% of all deaths

average age = 84.5

male:female ratio = 33:67

Atherosclerosis is a disease of the arterial blood vessels, often referred to as 'hardening' or 'furring' of the arteries, but the arteries to the heart and to the brain are excluded here.

See also Map 9 All cardiovascular deaths, Map 84 Heart attack and chronic heart disease and Map 98 Cerebrovascular disease.

From Plymouth, up along the Welsh coast, to Lancashire and the west of Scotland, rates are raised along this western edge of the island of Britain. To balance this, they are remarkably lower right down the eastern coast, from Aberdeen, through Dundee, much of Edinburgh, almost all of Leeds, and the bulk of the East Midlands and Birmingham; in western and northern Inner London, rates are below half the national average. Whether atherosclerosis or other diseases within the category of cardiovascular conditions gets coded on a death certificate may be largely arbitrary.

When atherosclerosis affects the arteries to the heart, it causes heart attacks and chronic heart disease. When it affects the arteries to the brain it causes cerebrovascular disease or strokes. The main arteries affected here are to the legs.

When the arteries harden they become narrower, restricting the supply of blood to organs of the body which can cause them to stop functioning properly. If the body's tissue does not receive a constant blood supply it can become infected and gangrene can develop.

Arteries are more likely to harden when a person eats a high fat diet, smokes, has diabetes and high blood pressure; moderate consumption of alcohol is thought to act against the development of atherosclerosis.

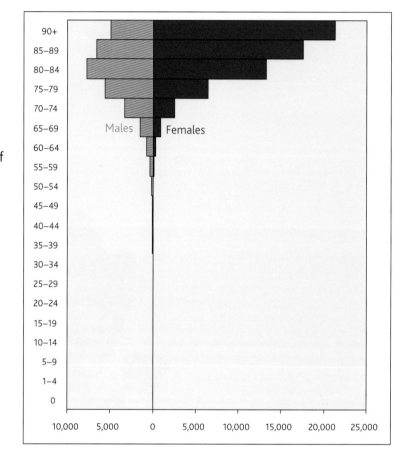

ICD-9 codes: 440
ICD-10 codes: I70

ICD-9	ICD-9 name	% of cases	ICD-10	ICD-10 name	% of cases
440	Atherosclerosis	100.0	I70	Atherosclerosis	100.0
		100.0			100.0

MAP 108 ATHEROSCLEROSIS

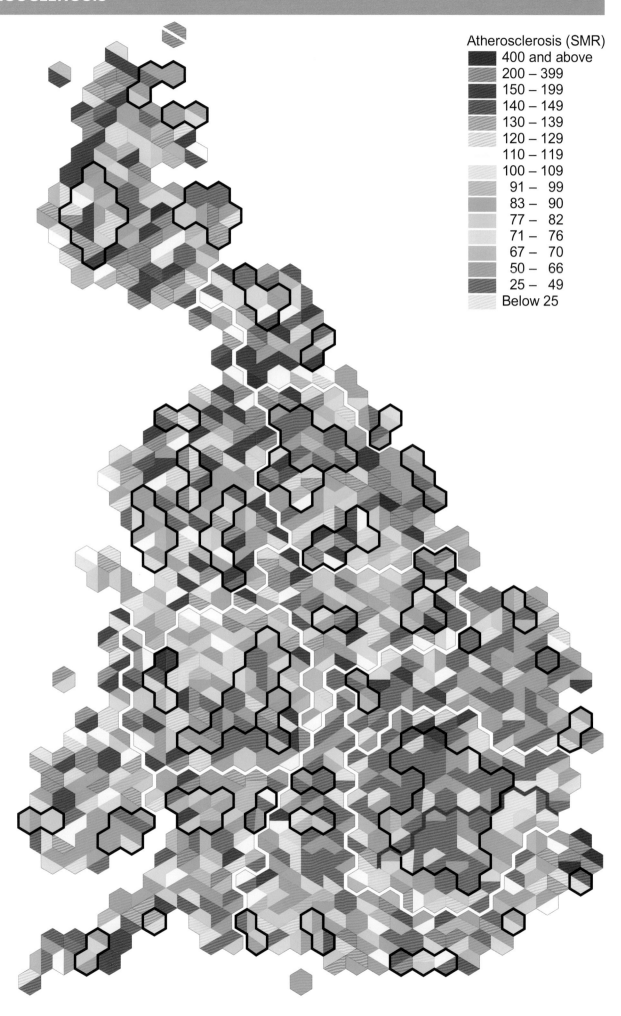

Atherosclerosis (SMR)

■	400 and above
▨	200 – 399
▨	150 – 199
▨	140 – 149
▨	130 – 139
▨	120 – 129
	110 – 119
	100 – 109
▨	91 – 99
▨	83 – 90
▨	77 – 82
▨	71 – 76
▨	67 – 70
▨	50 – 66
▨	25 – 49
▨	Below 25

109 OLD AGE

This cause of death includes those who are deemed to have died from 'senility without mention of psychosis', that is, old age without suffering from dementia.

152,564 cases

1.03% of all deaths

average age = 91.2

male:female ratio = 19:81

Death is not attributed to 'old age' in most of Scotland and the north and mid Wales. In contrast, in Hereford and Worcestershire, east Yorkshire, and north Devon it is much more commonly recorded. (Remember that our statistics take into account the age of the population in all the area and so the map does *not* reflect where more old people live, rather it reflects what they are considered to have died from.)

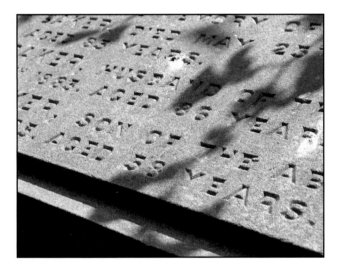

If ever you wished to see an example of how the last label that is given to us – the label of our cause of death – may be a little arbitrary in nature, it is through the geography of those deaths attributed to old age that geographical variation in cultural norms of certification of death becomes clear.

In these people who have been certified as dying of old age, post-mortem would show the most common cause of death to be pneumonia, but other infections, a silent (painless) heart attack or other condition might be found which had not been apparent. Many doctors will put down the most likely cause: pneumonia. Some will put down old age. Few would insist on a post-mortem at this age.

With the highest average age of death, at 91.2 years, to die of old age without senility is to die well.

ICD-9 codes: 797
ICD-10 codes: R54

ICD-9	ICD-9 name	% of cases	ICD-10	ICD-10 name	% of cases
797	Senility without mention of psychosis	100.0	R54	Senility	100.0
		100.0			100.0

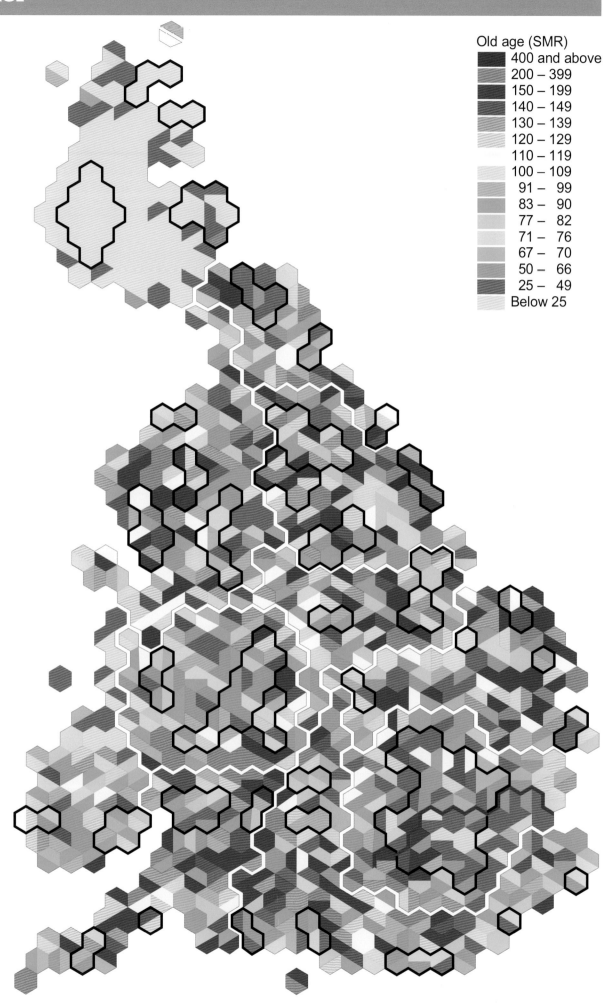

MAP 109   OLD AGE

Old age (SMR)
- 400 and above
- 200 – 399
- 150 – 199
- 140 – 149
- 130 – 139
- 120 – 129
- 110 – 119
- 100 – 109
- 91 – 99
- 83 – 90
- 77 – 82
- 71 – 76
- 67 – 70
- 50 – 66
- 25 – 49
- Below 25

Location appendix

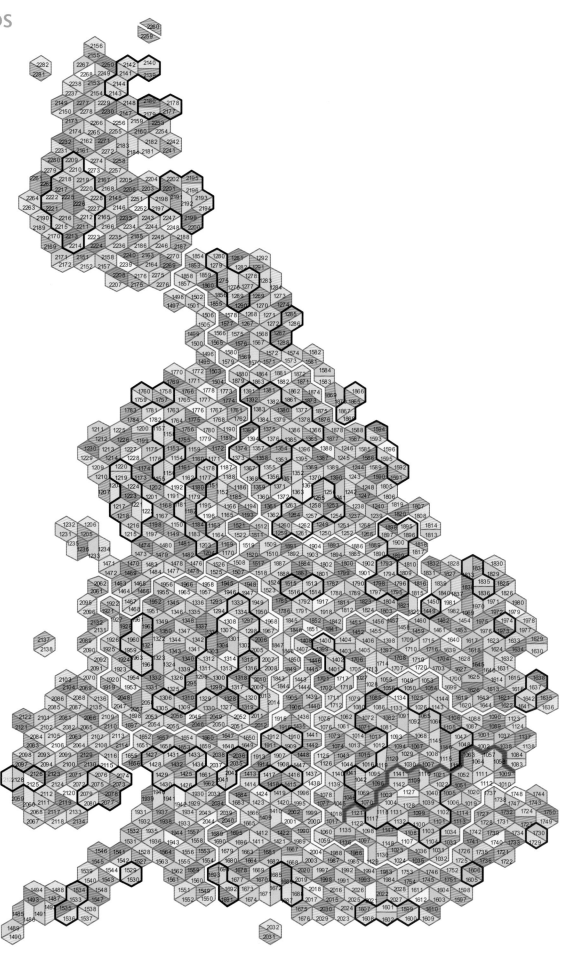

223

Number	Neighbourhood	Number	Neighbourhood	Number	Neighbourhood
1001	Barking North	1055	Cockfosters	1109	Southwark North
1002	Barking South	1056	Palmers Green	1110	Bermondsey
1003	Battersea West	1057	Abbey Wood	1111	East Wickham
1004	Battersea East	1058	Erith	1112	Sidcup
1005	Beckenham West	1059	Feltham	1113	Orpington West
1006	Beckenham East	1060	Heston	1114	Orpington East
1007	Stepney	1061	Golders Green	1115	Poplar
1008	Bow	1062	Finchley	1116	Canning Town
1009	Bexleyheath	1063	Greenwich	1117	Putney West
1010	Crayford	1064	Woolwich	1118	Putney East
1011	Cricklewood	1065	Stoke Newington	1119	Kensal Town
1012	Brondesbury	1066	Hackney North	1120	Regent's Park
1013	Sudbury (London)	1067	Shoreditch	1121	Richmond North
1014	Queensbury (London)	1068	Hackney South	1122	Richmond South
1015	Wembley	1069	Hammersmith	1123	Romford West
1016	Harlesden	1070	Fulham	1124	Romford East
1017	Isleworth	1071	Kilburn	1125	West Ruislip
1018	Brentford	1072	Highgate	1126	East Ruislip
1019	Bromley	1073	Harrow Weald	1127	Streatham North
1020	Chislehurst	1074	Greenhill	1128	Streatham South
1021	Camberwell Green	1075	Pinner	1129	Cheam
1022	Peckham	1076	Rayners Lane	1130	Sutton
1023	Carshalton	1077	Harlington	1131	Tooting West
1024	Wallington	1078	Hayes	1132	Tooting East
1025	Chingford	1079	Mill Hill	1133	Tottenham South
1026	Woodford Green	1080	Colindale	1134	Tottenham North
1027	Barnet West	1081	Holborn	1135	Twickenham North
1028	Barnet East	1082	St. Pancras	1136	Twickenham South
1029	Hyde Park	1083	Rainham	1137	Upminster North
1030	London Central	1084	Hacton	1138	Upminster South
1031	Croydon Addiscombe	1085	Fortis Green	1139	Uxbridge South
1032	Croydon Addington	1086	Hornsey	1140	Uxbridge North
1033	Selhurst	1087	Barkingside	1141	Vauxhall North
1034	Norwood	1088	Hainault	1142	Vauxhall South
1035	Coulsdon	1089	Loxford	1143	Walthamstow West
1036	Waddon	1090	Seven Kings	1144	Walthamstow East
1037	Dagenham West	1091	Tollington	1145	Forest Gate
1038	Dagenham East	1092	Highbury	1146	Plaistow
1039	West Norwood	1093	Holloway	1147	Wimbledon North
1040	Dulwich	1094	Canonbury	1148	Wimbledon South
1041	Acton	1095	Kensington	1149	Altrincham
1042	Shepherd's Bush	1096	Chelsea	1150	Sale West
1043	Greenford	1097	Surbiton	1151	Ashton West
1044	Ealing Broadway	1098	Kingston	1152	Ashton East
1045	Southall West	1099	Deptford North	1153	Bradshaw
1046	Southall East	1100	Deptford South	1154	Bolton Central
1047	East Ham North	1101	Grove Park	1155	Bolton Daubhill
1048	East Ham South	1102	Blackheath	1156	Little Lever
1049	Lower Edmonton	1103	Sydenham	1157	Horwich
1050	Upper Edmonton	1104	Catford	1158	Deane-Cum-Heaton
1051	Eltham West	1105	Leyton	1159	Tottington
1052	Eltham East	1106	Wanstead	1160	Bury Central
1053	Enfield Town	1107	Morden	1161	Radcliffe
1054	Enfield Highway	1108	Mitcham	1162	Prestwich

Number	Neighbourhood	Number	Neighbourhood	Number	Neighbourhood
1163	Cheadle Hulme	1217	Liverpool Riverside North	1271	Washington East
1164	Bramhall	1218	Liverpool Riverside South	1272	Houghton
1165	Reddish	1219	Walton South	1273	Jarrow North
1166	Denton	1220	Walton North	1274	Jarrow South
1167	Irlam	1221	Wavertree West	1275	Newcastle Fenham
1168	Swinton	1222	Wavertree East	1276	Newcastle Jesmond
1169	Romiley	1223	West Derby West	1277	Newcastle East
1170	Marple	1224	West Derby East	1278	Wallsend
1171	Middleton	1225	Rainford	1279	Newcastle Newburn
1172	Heywood	1226	Newton-Le-Willows	1280	Newcastle Dinnington
1173	Leigh South	1227	St. Helens Eccleston	1281	Longbenton
1174	Leigh North	1228	St. Helens Sutton	1282	Howdon
1175	Makerfield West	1229	Southport West	1283	South Shields West
1176	Makerfield East	1230	Southport East	1284	South Shields East
1177	Blackley South	1231	Wallasey West	1285	Southwick
1178	Blackley North	1232	Wallasey East	1286	Sunderland Central
1179	Moss Side	1233	Bebington	1287	South Hylton
1180	Ardwick	1234	Wirral Bromborough	1288	Sunderland Hendon
1181	Gorton West	1235	Hoylake	1289	Tyne Bridge West
1182	Gorton East	1236	Wirral Upton	1290	Tyne Bridge East
1183	Didsbury	1237	Barnsley Ardsley	1291	North Shields
1184	Burnage	1238	Barnsley Cudworth	1292	Whitley Bay
1185	Oldham East	1239	Barnsley East	1293	Brownhills
1186	Saddleworth	1240	Mexborough	1294	Aldridge
1187	Royton	1241	Penistone	1295	Edgbaston West
1188	Oldham West	1242	Barnsley West	1296	Edgbaston East
1189	Rochdale South	1243	Doncaster Town	1297	Erdington West
1190	Rochdale North	1244	Doncaster Armthorpe	1298	Erdington East
1191	Salford West	1245	Doncaster Adwick	1299	Hall Green West
1192	Salford East	1246	Doncaster Stainforth	1300	Hall Green East
1193	Hyde	1247	Don Valley West	1301	Hodge Hill West
1194	Stalybridge	1248	Don Valley East	1302	Hodge Hill East
1195	Stockport West	1249	Anston	1303	Ladywood West
1196	Stockport East	1250	Maltby	1304	Ladywood East
1197	Urmston	1251	Rotherham West	1305	Longbridge
1198	Stretford	1252	Rotherham East	1306	Northfield
1199	Wigan South	1253	Darnall	1307	Handsworth
1200	Wigan North	1254	Mosborough	1308	Oscott
1201	Tyldesley	1255	Owlerton	1309	Bournville
1202	Walkden	1256	Firth Park	1310	Moseley
1203	Sale East	1257	Sheffield City West	1311	Fox Hollies
1204	Wythenshawe	1258	Sheffield City East	1312	Sparkbrook
1205	Birkenhead South-West	1259	Hallam Moors	1313	Yardley West
1206	Birkenhead North-East	1260	Ecclesall	1314	Yardley East
1207	Bootle West	1261	Norton	1315	Coventry Longford
1208	Bootle East	1262	Intake	1316	Coventry Wyken
1209	Crosby North	1263	Stocksbridge	1317	Coventry Allesley
1210	Crosby South	1264	Walkley	1318	Coventry Radford
1211	Sefton East	1265	Wentworth West	1319	Coventry Earlsdon
1212	Knowsley North	1266	Wentworth East	1320	Coventry Cheylesmore
1213	Huyton	1267	Blaydon West	1321	Gornal
1214	Halewood	1268	Blaydon East	1322	Dudley Castle
1215	Garston South	1269	Gateshead East	1323	Kingswinford
1216	Garston North	1270	Washington West	1324	Brierley Hill

Number	Neighbourhood	Number	Neighbourhood	Number	Neighbourhood
1325	Halesowen	1379	Chapel Allerton	1433	Kingswood West
1326	Rowley	1380	Roundhay	1434	Kingswood East
1327	Meriden South	1381	Otley	1435	Aylesbury Rural
1328	Meriden North	1382	Headingley	1436	Aylesbury Urban
1329	Solihull West	1383	Kirkstall	1437	Beaconsfield West
1330	Solihull East	1384	Armley	1438	Beaconsfield East
1331	Stourbridge South	1385	Morley	1439	Buckingham West
1332	Stourbridge North	1386	Rothwell	1440	Buckingham East
1333	Sutton West	1387	Ossett	1441	Chesham
1334	Sutton East	1388	Stanley (Yorkshire)	1442	Amersham
1335	Willenhall	1389	Castleford	1443	Milton Keynes West
1336	Bloxwich	1390	Pontefract	1444	Bletchley
1337	Darlaston	1391	Pudsey North	1445	Milton Keynes North
1338	Walsall Paddock	1392	Pudsey South	1446	Newport Pagnell
1339	Warley West	1393	Bingley	1447	Wycombe Rural
1340	Warley East	1394	Baildon	1448	Wycombe Urban
1341	West Bromwich Central	1395	Denby Dale	1449	Cambridge West
1342	Great Barr	1396	Wakefield Central	1450	Cambridge East
1343	Oldbury	1397	Bedford West	1451	Huntingdon West
1344	Wednesbury	1398	Bedford East	1452	Huntingdon East
1345	Bushbury	1399	Luton Leagrave	1453	Littleport
1346	Wednesfield	1400	Luton Brambury	1454	Whittlesey
1347	Blakenhall	1401	Luton High Town	1455	Yaxley
1348	Bilston	1402	Caddington	1456	Orton
1349	Tettenhall	1403	Flitwick	1457	Peterborough West
1350	Graiseley	1404	Ampthill	1458	Peterborough East
1351	Spen	1405	East Bedfordshire	1459	Great Shelford
1352	Batley	1406	North Bedfordshire	1460	Hardwick
1353	Undercliffe	1407	Leighton Buzzard	1461	Fulbourn
1354	Eccleshill	1408	Dunstable	1462	Ely
1355	Queensbury (Bradford)	1409	Bracknell Forest	1463	Chester North
1356	Tong	1410	Bracknell Town	1464	Chester South
1357	Thornton	1411	Maidenhead West	1465	Congleton North
1358	Bradford University	1412	Maidenhead East	1466	Congleton South
1359	Todmorden	1413	Newbury Rural	1467	Crewe Urban
1360	Brighouse	1414	Newbury Urban	1468	Crewe Rural
1361	Marsden	1415	Reading Caversham	1469	Winsford Rural
1362	Holme Valley	1416	Reading North East	1470	Winsford Urban
1363	Dewsbury West	1417	Purley on Thames	1471	Ellesmere Port West
1364	Dewsbury East	1418	Reading Southcote	1472	Ellesmere Port East
1365	Garforth	1419	Slough West	1473	Runcorn
1366	Wetherby	1420	Slough East	1474	Widnes
1367	Halifax North	1421	Sunningdale	1475	Macclesfield Urban
1368	Halifax South	1422	Windsor and Eton	1476	Macclesfield Rural
1369	Featherstone	1423	Wokingham West	1477	Knutsford
1370	South Elmsall	1424	Wokingham East	1478	Wilmslow
1371	Huddersfield North	1425	Eastville	1479	Warrington Orford
1372	Huddersfield South	1426	Brislington	1480	Culcheth
1373	Keighley South	1427	Stoke Gifford	1481	Warrington Latchford
1374	Keighley North	1428	Avonmouth	1482	Lymm
1375	Leeds City	1429	Bedminster	1483	Weaver Vale North
1376	Hunslet	1430	Hengrove	1484	Weaver Vale South
1377	Harehills	1431	Clifton	1485	Camborne
1378	Halton	1432	Redland	1486	Falmouth

Number	Neighbourhood	Number	Neighbourhood	Number	Neighbourhood
1487	Newquay	1541	Tiverton	1595	Hessle
1488	North Cornwall Rural	1542	Honiton	1596	Hull West
1489	Penzance	1543	Paignton	1597	Bexhill
1490	Helston	1544	Torquay	1598	Battle
1491	St. Blazey	1545	West Devon	1599	Brighton East
1492	Torpoint	1546	Torridge	1600	Peacehaven
1493	Truro	1547	Totnes West	1601	Brighton West
1494	St. Austell	1548	Totnes East	1602	Brighton Central
1495	Barrow-in-Furness	1549	Bournemouth Moordown	1603	Eastbourne West
1496	Ulverston	1550	Bournemouth Boscombe	1604	Eastbourne East
1497	Carlisle West	1551	Bournemouth Kinson	1605	Hastings West
1498	Carlisle East	1552	Bournemouth Central	1606	Hastings East
1499	Whitehaven	1553	Christchurch North-West	1607	Hove Inland
1500	Copeland Rural	1554	Christchurch South-East	1608	Hove Coast
1501	Penrith Urban	1555	Mid Dorset	1609	Lewes South
1502	Penrith Rural	1556	Poole North	1610	Lewes North
1503	Westmorland Rural	1557	North West Dorset	1611	Crowborough
1504	Westmorland Urban	1558	North East Dorset	1612	Hailsham
1505	Workington West	1559	Poole Town	1613	Stanford Le Hope
1506	Workington East	1560	Poole Branksome	1614	Basildon Central
1507	Amber Valley West	1561	Weymouth	1615	Billericay West
1508	Amber Valley East	1562	Swanage	1616	Billericay East
1509	Clowne	1563	West Dorset Rural	1617	Braintree North-West
1510	Shirebrook	1564	West Dorset Urban	1618	Braintree South East
1511	Chesterfield West	1565	Barnard Castle	1619	Chipping Ongar
1512	Chesterfield East	1566	Spennymoor	1620	Brentwood
1513	Allestree	1567	Durham City South	1621	Benfleet
1514	Chaddesden	1568	Durham City North	1622	Canvey Island
1515	Mickleover	1569	Darlington West	1623	Colchester West
1516	Alvaston	1570	Darlington East	1624	Colchester East
1517	Ilkeston	1571	Peterlee	1625	Epping
1518	Long Eaton	1572	Seaham	1626	Chigwell
1519	Glossop	1573	Hartlepool West	1627	Harlow West
1520	Buxton	1574	Hartlepool East	1628	Harlow East
1521	Dronfield	1575	Stanley (Durham)	1629	Harwich North
1522	Clay Cross	1576	Chester-Le-Street	1630	Harwich South
1523	Swadlincote	1577	Crook	1631	Chelmsford East
1524	Repton	1578	Consett	1632	Maldon
1525	Belper	1579	Sedgefield West	1633	North West Essex
1526	Matlock	1580	Sedgefield East	1634	North East Essex
1527	Exmouth	1581	Stockton Norton	1635	Rayleigh West
1528	East Devon Rural	1582	Billingham	1636	Rayleigh East
1529	Exeter West	1583	Eaglescliffe	1637	Southend East
1530	Exeter East	1584	Stockton Fairfield	1638	Rochford
1531	North Devon Rural	1585	Beverley	1639	Saffron Walden West
1532	North Devon Urban	1586	North Humberside Coast	1640	Saffron Walden East
1533	Plymouth North-West	1587	East Yorkshire Rural	1641	Southend Leigh
1534	Plymouth North-East	1588	East Yorkshire Coast	1642	Southend Prittlewell
1535	Plymouth Peverell	1589	Howden	1643	Thurrock West
1536	Plymouth Waterfront	1590	Cottingham	1644	Thurrock East
1537	Plympton	1591	Sutton-On-Hull	1645	Chelmsford Rural West
1538	Ivybridge	1592	Hull Marfleet	1646	Chelmsford Moulsham
1539	Teignbridge Rural	1593	Hull University	1647	Cheltenham North
1540	Teignbridge Urban	1594	Hull Bransholme	1648	Cheltenham South

Number	Neighbourhood	Number	Neighbourhood	Number	Neighbourhood
1649	Cotswold South West	1703	Hertford	1757	Blackpool North
1650	Cotswold North East	1704	Bishop's Stortford	1758	Fleetwood
1651	Forest of Dean Urban	1705	Bushey	1759	Blackpool Marton
1652	Forest of Dean Rural	1706	Borehamwood	1760	Blackpool South Shore
1653	Gloucester West	1707	Harpenden	1761	Burnley West
1654	Gloucester East	1708	Hitchin	1762	Burnley East
1655	Chipping Sodbury West	1709	Letchworth	1763	Chorley Rural
1656	Chipping Sodbury East	1710	North-East Hertfordshire Rural	1764	Chorley Urban
1657	Stroud Rural	1711	West Hertfordshire	1765	Lytham St. Anne's
1658	Stroud Urban	1712	South Hertfordshire	1766	Kirkham
1659	Tewkesbury South-West	1713	St. Albans West	1767	Great Harwood
1660	Tewkesbury North-East	1714	St. Albans East	1768	Accrington
1661	Keynsham	1715	Stevenage North	1769	Poulton-le-Fylde
1662	Norton-Radstock	1716	Stevenage South	1770	Lancaster
1663	Aldershot North	1717	Watford Outer	1771	Morecambe
1664	Aldershot South	1718	Watford Central	1772	Carnforth
1665	Basingstoke West	1719	Welwyn Garden City	1773	Barnoldswick
1666	Basingstoke East	1720	Hatfield	1774	Nelson
1667	Petersfield	1721	Ashford Urban	1775	Preston South-West
1668	Horndean	1722	Ashford Rural	1776	Preston East
1669	Eastleigh North	1723	Canterbury South	1777	Preston North
1670	Eastleigh South	1724	Canterbury North	1778	Clitheroe
1671	Fareham West	1725	Aylesford	1779	Darwen
1672	Fareham East	1726	Chatham	1780	Rawtenstall
1673	Gosport West	1727	Dartford South	1781	Preston Middleforth
1674	Gosport East	1728	Dartford North	1782	Leyland
1675	Havant Central	1729	Dover West	1783	Ormskirk
1676	Hayling and Emsworth	1730	Dover East	1784	Skelmersdale
1677	Lyndhurst	1731	Maidstone East	1785	Lutterworth
1678	Totton	1732	Faversham	1786	Narborough
1679	Ringwood	1733	Folkestone Rural	1787	Bosworth West
1680	New Milton	1734	Folkestone Urban	1788	Bosworth East
1681	Fleet	1735	Gillingham West	1789	Charnwood West
1682	Bordon	1736	Gillingham East	1790	Charnwood East
1683	Andover	1737	Northfleet	1791	Wigston
1684	Whitchurch	1738	Gravesend	1792	Market Harborough
1685	Portsmouth Cosham	1739	Maidstone West	1793	Belgrave
1686	Portsmouth Drayton	1740	The Weald	1794	Evington
1687	Portsea	1741	Medway South	1795	Aylestone
1688	Milton	1742	Medway North	1796	Knighton
1689	Romsey Rural	1743	Herne Bay	1797	North Braunstone
1690	Romsey Urban	1744	Margate	1798	Beaumont Leys
1691	Southampton Bitterne	1745	Sevenoaks South	1799	Loughborough West
1692	Southampton Sholing	1746	Sevenoaks North	1800	Loughborough East
1693	Southampton Millbrook	1747	Sittingbourne	1801	Ashby de la Zouch
1694	Southampton Portswood	1748	Sheppey	1802	Castle Donington
1695	Winchester West	1749	Ramsgate Inland	1803	Boston
1696	Winchester East	1750	Ramsgate Coastal	1804	Skegness
1697	Hereford Rural	1751	Tonbridge	1805	Goole
1698	Hereford Urban	1752	Malling	1806	Brigg
1699	Cheshunt South	1753	Tunbridge Wells West	1807	Cleethorpes West
1700	Cheshunt North	1754	Tunbridge Wells East	1808	Cleethorpes East
1701	Hemel Hempstead West	1755	Blackburn West	1809	Gainsborough West
1702	Hemel Hempstead East	1756	Blackburn East	1810	Gainsborough East

Number	Neighbourhood	Number	Neighbourhood	Number	Neighbourhood
1973	Ipswich West	2027	Burgess Hill	2081	Carmarthen East Rural
1974	Ipswich East	2028	East Grinstead	2082	Carmarthen East Urban
1975	Sudbury (Suffolk)	2029	Worthing Rustington	2083	South Pembrokeshire
1976	Hadleigh	2030	Worthing Central	2084	Carmarthen West
1977	Suffolk Coastal South	2031	Isle of Wight West	2085	Ceredigion Urban
1978	Suffolk Coastal North	2032	Isle of Wight East	2086	Ceredigion Rural
1979	Waveney Rural	2033	Devizes Urban	2087	Cefn Mawr
1980	Lowestoft	2034	Devizes Rural	2088	Rhostyllen
1981	Mildenhall	2035	Swindon North	2089	Colwyn Bay
1982	Haverhill	2036	Swindon Rural	2090	Clwyd Rural
1983	Caterham	2037	Chippenham	2091	Bangor
1984	Oxted	2038	Wootton Bassett	2092	Llandudno
1985	Epsom	2039	Salisbury Rural	2093	Aberdare North
1986	Ewell	2040	Salisbury Urban	2094	Aberdare South
1987	Walton	2041	Swindon West	2095	Holywell
1988	Esher	2042	Swindon South-East	2096	Mold
1989	Guildford Rural	2043	Trowbridge	2097	Gower South West
1990	Guildford Urban	2044	Warminster	2098	Gower North East
1991	Dorking	2045	Bromsgrove Urban	2099	Blackwood
1992	Leatherhead	2046	Bromsgrove Rural	2100	Newbridge
1993	Reigate South	2047	Leominster Rural	2101	Llanelli Rural
1994	Reigate North	2048	Leominster Urban	2102	Llanelli Urban
1995	Weybridge	2049	Droitwich	2103	Meirionnydd Urban
1996	Addlestone	2050	Evesham	2104	Meirionnydd Rural
1997	Farnham	2051	Redditch South	2105	Merthyr Tydfil
1998	Godalming	2052	Redditch North	2106	Rhymney
1999	Staines	2053	Great Malvern Rural	2107	Monmouth Urban
2000	Sunbury	2054	Great Malvern Urban	2108	Monmouth Rural
2001	Surrey Heath South	2055	Worcester West	2109	Montgomeryshire Rural
2002	Surrey Heath North	2056	Worcester East	2110	Montgomeryshire Urban
2003	Woking West	2057	Wyre Forest Rural	2111	Neath Urban
2004	Woking East	2058	Wyre Forest Urban	2112	Neath Rural
2005	Bedworth	2059	Aberavon West	2113	Newport St. Julians
2006	Atherstone	2060	Aberavon East	2114	Caldicot
2007	Nuneaton West	2061	Buckley	2115	Rogerstone
2008	Nuneaton East	2062	Connah's Quay	2116	Newport Gaer
2009	Rugby Rural	2063	Ebbw Vale	2117	Maesteg
2010	Rugby Urban	2064	Brynmawr	2118	Aberkenfig
2011	Stratford-on-Avon West	2065	Brecon Urban	2119	Pontypridd West
2012	Stratford-on-Avon East	2066	Brecon Rural	2120	Pontypridd East
2013	Warwick	2067	Bridgend West	2121	Preseli Rural
2014	Leamington	2068	Bridgend East	2122	Preseli Urban
2015	Arundel	2069	Caernarfon Rural	2123	Rhondda North
2016	South Downs East	2070	Caernarfon Urban	2124	Rhondda South
2017	Bognor Regis	2071	Caerphilly North	2125	Swansea Landore
2018	Littlehampton	2072	Caerphilly South	2126	Swansea Llansamlet
2019	Chichester South	2073	Cardiff Cathays	2127	Killay
2020	Chichester North	2074	Cardiff Cyncoed	2128	Swansea Townhill
2021	Crawley West	2075	Tongwynlais	2129	Pontypool
2022	Crawley East	2076	Lisvane	2130	Cwmbran
2023	Worthing East	2077	Penarth	2131	Prestatyn and Ryhl
2024	Shoreham	2078	Cardiff South	2132	Saint Asaph
2025	Horsham Rural	2079	Cardiff Radyr	2133	Glamorgan Rural
2026	Horsham Urban	2080	Cardiff Ely	2134	Barry

Number	Neighbourhood	Number	Neighbourhood	Number	Neighbourhood
2135	Wrexham South-West	2185	East Kilbride North	2235	Blantyre
2136	Wrexham North-East	2186	East Kilbride South	2236	Hamilton Cadzow
2137	Anglesey West	2187	Prestonpans	2237	Mallaig
2138	Anglesey East	2188	Haddington	2238	Inverness East
2139	Aberdeen Queens Cross	2189	Barrhead	2239	Kilmarncock Central
2140	Old Aberdeen	2190	Giffnock	2240	Kilmarncock Rural
2141	Aberdeen West	2191	Edinburgh Murrayfield	2241	Kirkcaldy South
2142	Dyce	2192	Edinburgh Holyrood	2242	Kirkcaldy North
2143	Aberdeen South-West	2193	Edinburgh East	2243	Linlithgow North
2144	Aberdeen Nigg Bay	2194	Musselburgh	2244	Linlithgow South
2145	Airdrie	2195	Leith	2245	Livingston Central
2146	Shotts	2196	Edinburgh North	2246	Livingston Rural
2147	Sidlaw and Carnoustie	2197	Balerno	2247	Midlothian North-West
2148	Montrose and Arbroath	2198	Edinburgh Sighthill	2248	Midlothian South-East
2149	Lorn	2199	Edinburgh Morningside	2249	Forres
2150	Bute	2200	Edinburgh Kaimes	2250	Elgin
2151	Prestwick and Troon	2201	Queensferry	2251	Motherwell
2152	Ayr Central	2202	Edinburgh Corstorphine	2252	Wishaw
2153	Banff	2203	Falkirk Laurieston	2253	Newburgh
2154	Buchan	2204	Grangemouth	2254	St Andrews
2155	Caithness	2205	Denny	2255	Coupar Angus
2156	Wick	2206	Falkirk Central	2256	Forfar
2157	Carrick	2207	Stranraer	2257	Bridge of Allan
2158	Cumnock and Doon Valley	2208	Nithsdale	2258	Alloa
2159	Glenrothes	2209	Glasgow Blairdardie	2259	Orkney
2160	Leven	2210	Glasgow Knightswood	2260	Shetland
2161	Clydebank	2211	Glasgow Baillieston	2261	Linwood
2162	Milngavie	2212	Glasgow Easterhouse	2262	Paisley Gallowhill
2163	Larkhall	2213	Glasgow Newlands	2263	Johnstone
2164	Lanark	2214	Glasgow Castlemilk	2264	Paisley Blackhall
2165	Chryston	2215	Glasgow Pollokshields	2265	Crieff
2166	Coatbridge	2216	Glasgow Ibrox	2266	Perth Central
2167	Kilsyth	2217	Glasgow University	2267	Dingwall and Skye
2168	Cumbernauld	2218	Glasgow Partick	2268	Inverness West
2169	Saltcoats and Arran	2219	Glasgow Maryhill	2269	Roxburgh
2170	Largs and Cumbrae	2220	Glasgow Milton	2270	Berwickshire
2171	Kilwinning	2221	Glasgow Nitshill	2271	Stirling Rural
2172	Irvine	2222	Glasgow Cardonald	2272	Stirling Urban
2173	Helensburgh	2223	Rutherglen West	2273	Bearsden and Kirkintilloch South
2174	Dumbarton Central	2224	Rutherglen East	2274	Kirkintilloch North
2175	Dumfries Central	2225	Glasgow Calton	2275	Tweeddale
2176	Dumfries East	2226	Glasgow Parkhead	2276	Ettrick and Lauderdale
2177	Dundee South-East	2227	Glasgow Cowlairs	2277	Banchory
2178	Dundee North-East	2228	Glasgow Robroyston	2278	Stonehaven
2179	Dundee South-West	2229	Turriff	2279	Bridge of Weir
2180	Dundee North-West	2230	Inverurie	2280	Port Glasgow
2181	Dunfermline North-East	2231	Greenock South	2281	Eilean Siar Rural
2182	Cowdenbeath	2232	Greenock North	2282	Stornoway
2183	Dunfermline South-West	2233	Hamilton North		
2184	Dunfermline Central	2234	Belshill		

Technical appendix

ICD codes

The International Classification of Diseases (ICD), maintained by the World Health Organisation (WHO), is the international standard diagnostic classification. It is used for classifying both morbidity and mortality. The ICD is currently on its tenth revision (ICD-10); as advances in diagnoses occur and opinions change, it is periodically totally revised. The period covered by this atlas (1981 to 2004) spans two versions of the ICD, 9 and 10. A brief history of the classification can be found on the WHO website (www.who.int/classifications/icd/en/HistoryOfICD.pdf).

Additionally, updates within a revision can also be made. For example, there was originally no coding for MRSA (Methicillin-resistant *Staphylococcus aureus*) in ICD-10. However, as the incidence of MRSA has increased so much in recent years the WHO has added codes to identify it; however, this update was not applied until after the period that this atlas covers. Atlases of mortality usually map prevalent diseases defined according to contemporary medical categorisation.

Table 1: ICD-9 chapters

ICD-9 Chapter	Blocks	ICD-9 Title
I	001–139	Infectious and parasitic diseases
II	140–239	Neoplasm
III	240–279	Endocrine, nutritional and metabolic diseases and immunity disorders
IV	280–289	Diseases of the blood and blood forming organs
V	290–319	Mental disorders
VI	320–389	Diseases of the nervous system and sense organs
VII	390–459	Diseases of the circulatory system
VIII	460–519	Diseases of the respiratory system
IX	520–579	Diseases of the digestive system
X	580–629	Diseases of the genito-urinary system
XI	630–677	Complications pregnancy, childbirth and pueperium
XII	680–709	Diseases of the skin and subcutaneous tissue
XIII	710–739	Diseases of the musculoskeletal system and cognitive tissue
XIV	740–759	Congenital anomalies
XV	760–779	Certain conditions originating in the perinatal period
XVI	780–799	Symptoms, signs and ill-defined conditions
XVII	*800–999*	*Injury and poisoning*
E	E800–E999	Supplementary classification of external causes of injury and poisoning
Supp	*V01–V82*	*Supplementary classification of factors influencing health status and contact with health services*

Table 2: ICD-10 chapters

ICD-10 Chapter	Blocks	ICD-10 Title
I	A00-B99	Certain infectious and parasitic diseases
II	C00-D48	Neoplasms
III	D50-D89	Diseases of the blood and blood-forming organs and certain disorders involving the immune mechanism
IV	E00-E90	Endocrine, nutritional and metabolic diseases
V	F00-F99	Mental and behavioural disorders
VI	G00-G99	Diseases of the nervous system
VII	H00-H59	Diseases of the eye and adnexa
VIII	H60-H95	Diseases of the ear and mastoid process
IX	I00-I99	Diseases of the circulatory system
X	J00-J99	Diseases of the respiratory system
XI	K00-K93	Diseases of the digestive system
XII	L00-L99	Diseases of the skin and subcutaneous tissue
XIII	M00-M99	Diseases of the musculoskeletal system and connective tissue
XIV	N00-N99	Diseases of the genitourinary system
XV	O00-O99	Pregnancy, childbirth and the puerperium
XVI	P00-P96	Certain conditions originating in the perinatal period
XVII	Q00-Q99	Congenital malformations, deformations and chromosomal abnormalities
XVIII	R00-R99	Symptoms, signs and abnormal clinical and laboratory findings, not elsewhere classified
XIX	*S00-T98*	*Injury, poisoning and certain other consequences of external causes*
XX	V01-Y98	External causes of morbidity and mortality
XXI	*Z00-Z99*	*Factors influencing health status and contact with health services*

Note: Chapters in both ICD-9 and ICD-10 shown in italics are not used for classifying underlying cause of death in this atlas.

As can be seen from Table 1 of ICD-9 chapters and Table 2 of ICD-10 chapters, there are more chapters in ICD-10 than ICD-9; additionally some diseases have been moved from one chapter to another, reflecting changing medical opinion. Furthermore, there are more individual disease causes in ICD-10 than in ICD-9. Both classifications give a code for every named disease and cause of death.

Of more importance, however, was the change of rules for coding the underlying cause of death on the death certificate. The 'underlying cause of death', is defined by WHO as:

a) the disease or injury which initiated the train of events directly leading to death or
b) the circumstances of the accident or violence which produced the fatal injury.

Deaths were first coded to ICD-10 in Scotland in 2000 and in England and Wales in 2001. Note that the ICD versions as used by the registration agencies were used for the appropriate time periods here.

As a result of these changes, a significant condition contributing to the death, as entered in part II of the cause of death certificate, is now more often classified as the underlying cause of death than previously. This is particularly the case when the cause of death given in part I is commonly given as the eventual cause of death for people suffering from a chronic progressive disease given in part II which has been of long duration.

The change is expected to cause the classification of deaths as due to pneumonia (when often thought of as a merciful release) to fall by 40%. Deaths now classified as due to mental disorder and due to musculoskeletal disease are both expected to be about 40% higher due to the different classification rules. In particular, deaths from Alzheimer's disease (included in Other nervous disorders) will double and those from Parkinson's disease will increase by 50%. The more recent figures are included in our statistics without any adjustment, but are unlikely to affect the appearance of the map. Further details can be found at www.statistics.gov.uk/about/classifications/icd10/default.asp.

Our categories are usually based on ICD-9 and we used the mapping from ICD-10 to ICD-9 obtained from: www.health.gov.au/internet/main/publishing.nsf/content/health-casemix-mapdis1.htm to include the most recent deaths. The tables in each section of the atlas show the individual ICD-9 and ICD-10 codes that make up each category and the proportions of deaths for each code. Note that ICD codes are hierarchical, so, for example, ICD-9 002 is the sum of 002.0 to 002.9, and ICD-10

A01 is the sum of A01.0 to A01.9. The last category is frequently 'other something' meaning all of the next level up except those conditions already specified at the current level.

Registration of death

It is a legal requirement that deaths are registered with the General Register Office for deaths occurring in England and Wales and with the General Register Office for Scotland for deaths occurring in Scotland.

Figure 1 shows an example of a death certificate.

The rules regarding the usual residence of a deceased person living in an institution have changed over time. Up to 1992, for those living in residential homes, this was considered to be their usual residence – even if they had been there for only one day. From 1958 to 1992 there was a six-month residency rule for residents of chronic sick and psychiatric hospitals, and from 1980 also for residents of geriatric hospitals. However, from 1993, it has been up to the informant registering the death to decide the deceased's usual residence (see Office for National Statistics (2000), *Review of the Registrar General on deaths in England and Wales, 1998*, London: The Stationery Office for details).

At registration of death, informants can choose which address to use. So, for example, the parents of a boy who was a pupil at Eton College would probably register his home address as his usual residence. Similarly, when registering the death of his 20-year-old sister, a student at Manchester University, it is likely that they would also use the home address as her usual residence.

Figure 1: Example of a death certificate

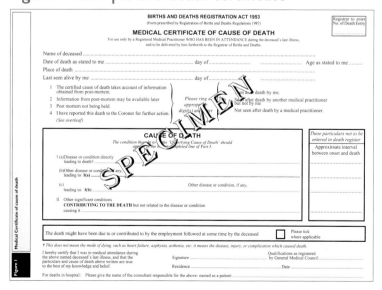

Source: www.statistics.gov.uk/about/Classifications/ICD10/downloads/Death_Certificate.pdf

Over the course of time that this project covered, different parts of the country changed over from the ninth to the tenth revision of the ICD system at different dates and we had to allow for that and use both coding systems in this atlas. Note also that no additional adjustments have been made here to allow for any accompanying rule changes; we used the code that was in the original data. The effects are, for instance, that more deaths were coded to pneumonia under the old system, fewer under the new, but the effects on maps that cover 24 years and which do not attempt to show changing rates over time are small.

Most undetermined deaths (open verdicts) among adults are cases where the harm is likely to have been self-inflicted and intentionally self-inflicted but there was insufficient evidence to prove that the deceased deliberately intended to killed themselves (Charlton, J., Kelly, S., Dunnell, K., Evans, B., Jenkins, R. and Wallis, R. (1992) 'Trends in suicide deaths in England and Wales', *Population Trends*, no 69, pp 10–16, London: HMSO).

Data and geography

Mortality data were supplied with postcodes for England and Wales by the Office for National Statistics (ONS), and with postcode sectors for Scotland by the General Register Office for Scotland (GRO(S)). For the relevant time period, they have been georeferenced (defined in physical space and entered into a Geographical Information System) to the ward (or equivalent) extant at the time of the preceding Census:

Mortality 1981–1990 = 1981 Census Wards in England & Wales, Postcode Sectors in Scotland

Mortality 1991–2000 = 1991 Census Wards in England & Wales, Postcode Sectors in Scotland

Mortality 2001–2004 = 2001 Standard Table (ST) Wards in England, ST Electoral Divisions in Wales and ST Postcode Sectors in Scotland.

For convenience we refer to all of these as 'wards'.

However, as we are looking at a period of 24 years, there have been numerous ward boundary changes and we need to use a geography that takes these into account. Therefore we have used neighbourhoods, which are aggregations of wards such that geographical change over time is minimised (Further details can be found in SASI (2006), 'Tracts Information', Social and Spatial Inequalities Research Group, University of Sheffield, www.sasi. group.shef.ac.uk/tracts). Additionally, neighbourhoods were

designed to have as equal-sized population as possible. Each of the 1,282 neighbourhoods is approximately half a Westminster parliamentary constituency as they stood at the 2001 General Election. A further reason for using a larger geography than wards is the need to maintain confidentiality. No single death can be identified, and aggregating to a larger geography allows this to be achieved.

Population

We have mortality data for a 24-year period from 1981 to 2004. To calculate rates and ratios we needed to estimate a population at risk of death figure to cover this period: as the population of Great Britain has changed over this period we need to reflect these changes. The model we used was

Population = ((1981 population * 5) + (1991 population * 10) + (2001 population * 9))

This comes to 24 years of figures suitably weighted. However, for a variety of reasons we cannot just use the census population figures as published.

1981 population figures

We used data from the 1981 Census Table 2 All Residents. Unfortunately this table has the youngest age group as 0–4 and does not distinguish infants under the age of 1. Therefore, to calculate the number of infants aged 0 and the number of children aged 1–4, we took the proportion of 0 year olds of 0–4 year olds from children in households (Census Table 25) and applied that to all 0–4 year olds to get a figure for 0 year olds, and by subtraction, 1–4 year olds.

The 1981 Census only goes up to age 85+, while we wanted figures for 85–89 and 90+. After trying a variety of models, and checking against the Government Actuary's national population projections, the best fit was to apply the 1991 Census proportion that those aged 90+ comprised of those aged 85+ to the 1981 data.

1991 population figures

We had originally planned to use the Estimating with Confidence (EwC) 1991 figures for our 1991 population (www.ccsr.ac.uk/research/ewcpop.htm). However, following the 2001 Census it was generally realised that although the original 1991

Census figures were too low, the EwC figures were possibly too high. Paul Norman and colleagues (Norman, P., Simpson, L. and Sabater, A. (submitted), 'Estimating with confidence and hindsight: new UK small area population estimates for 1991', *Population, Space & Place*) have calculated revised EwC figures, and this is what we chose to use.

The revised EwC data has the same problems with age bands at each extreme as 1981; the same solutions were applied.

2001 population figures

The 2001 population figures were taken from 2001 Census Standard Table 001.

Putting the students back home

Both the 1991 revised EwC and the 2001 Census put students at their term-time address and not at their home address. Mortality rates for young people are low so it might be thought that this was unimportant. However, young people at university are concentrated in small geographical areas. Further, in some places students tend to live in the poorer parts of town (where there are higher mortality rates) and their large numbers would have a huge effect on rates there; this is compounded by the fact that for those who do die, their parents are likely to register their usual residence as being their home address. Therefore, we have to put the students back home.

The 1991 revised EwC includes a student adjustment (putting students in college) so it was simple to reverse this adjustment to put them back at their home address.

For 2001, we commissioned from the ONS and GRO(S) two census tables at neighbourhood geography. The first was Table ST012 *Schoolchildren and Students in Full-Time Education Living Away From Home in Term-Time by Age*. This table tells us, by sex and age, the number of schoolchildren and students who would be living in the area were they not away at an educational establishment; this gives us the number of people to add in. The second commissioned table (Table 3) was of the *Accommodation* variables for Table TT002 *Students and Schoolchildren*. This table tells us in what type of accommodation schoolchildren and students are living:

We then developed two models, one for schoolchildren aged 10–18 and one for students aged 19 and over.

Table 3: Accommodation variables for students and schoolchildren

Living in a household:
Student living alone
Living in parent(s) household
All student group household
Other household
Living in a communal establishment:
Educational establishment
Other communal establishment

For schoolchildren (aged 10–18) we took the sum of children not living with parents or in other households. We assumed that children in other households are living with another relative or with foster parents and are in fact in their home neighbourhood. Then we multiplied this by some proportion, x, such that the total number taken away equals the total number that needs to be added in.

Revised Population = Census Population + Students Away − ((Educational Establishment + Other Communal Establishment + All Student Group Households + Students Living Alone) * x)

Note that x varies by sex and age, the age bands being under 10, 10–11, 12-14, 15, 16, 17, and 18. Note also that this method does not take into account the number of schoolchildren who live in the same neighbourhood where they are at school. For example, a boy whose parents live in Windsor and who boards at Eton would be subtracted but not added in the formula above.

The model for students aged over 18 was slightly different:

Revised Population = Census Population + Students Away − ((Educational Establishment + Other Communal Establishment + All Student Group Households + Students Living Alone + Other Households) * x)

Again, x varies by sex and age; here the age bands were 19, 20, 21, 22, 23, 24, 25-29, 30-34 and 35+.

Finally, we put the revised population, by sex, into the 5-year bands 10–14, 15–19, 20-24 and 25–29. The calculations for the under 10s and over 29s were so close to the original census figures that we decided to use the latter.

Because we applied a global proportion for each sex and age, some neighbourhoods may be better dealt with than others.

Indirect SMR

Because age and sex has a bearing on what we die of, we cannot just use crude death rates to explain patterns of mortality as different neighbourhoods have different age–sex population structures. Therefore we used *indirect* age–sex standardised mortality ratios (SMRs).

$$SMR = \frac{Observed\ deaths\ in\ neighbourhood}{Expected\ deaths\ in\ neighbourhood} * 100$$

We calculated the national age–sex specific rates for each cause of death for the national population.

These national rates were then multiplied by the population of each neighbourhood for each age band across both sexes and for all people. This gave us the expected number of deaths from each cause in each neighbourhood if they conformed to the national average. We used the indirect ratio because the direct ratio is not well specified when no deaths occur for a particular cause for a particular age and sex group over the course of the 24 years mapped here.

Finally, we divided the observed number of deaths in each neighbourhood by the expected number of deaths and multiplied by 100 to arrive at the indirect SMR. An SMR of 100 means that there is no difference between the observed and the expected number of deaths. An SMR over 100 means that mortality is higher – for example an SMR of 120 means that mortality is 20% higher than that of the general population, and an SMR below 100 means that mortality in that neighbourhood is lower than average.

Because we are mapping deaths over a 24-year period for areas with an average population of about 40,000 people we have not smoothed the results but show actual ratios that occurred. We have also not attempted to give an indication of the numbers of deaths involved simultaneously with the ratios as this would be extremely confusing cartographically. However, we do give advice in the introduction of this atlas as to the interpretation of patterns based on a national total of less than 5,000 deaths. The number of deaths being mapped is shown opposite each map.

Table 4a: Most common and second most common cause of death at each age band – males

Males age	Most common cause of death	Second most common cause of death
0	Conditions of the perinatal period	Sudden death, cause unknown
1–4	Congenital heart defects	Other nervous disorders
5–9	Pedestrian hit by vehicle	Leukaemia
10–14	Pedestrian hit by vehicle	Other nervous disorders
15–19	Motor vehicle accidents	Suicide/undetermined intent by hanging
20–24	Motor vehicle accidents	Suicide/undetermined intent by hanging
25–29	Motor vehicle accidents	Deaths due to drugs
30–34	Motor vehicle accidents	Suicide/undetermined intent by hanging
35–39	Heart attack and chronic heart disease	Suicide/undetermined intent by hanging
40–44	Heart attack and chronic heart disease	Chronic liver disease
45–49	Heart attack and chronic heart disease	Lung cancer
50–54	Heart attack and chronic heart disease	Lung cancer
55–59	Heart attack and chronic heart disease	Lung cancer
60–64	Heart attack and chronic heart disease	Lung cancer
65–69	Heart attack and chronic heart disease	Lung cancer
70–74	Heart attack and chronic heart disease	Lung cancer
75–79	Heart attack and chronic heart disease	Cerebrovascular disease
80–84	Heart attack and chronic heart disease	Cerebrovascular disease
85–89	Heart attack and chronic heart disease	Cerebrovascular disease
90+	Heart attack and chronic heart disease	Pneumonia

Table 4b: Most common and second most common cause of death at each age band – females

Females age	Most common cause of death	Second most common cause of death
0	Conditions of the perinatal period	Sudden death, cause unknown
1–4	Congenital heart defects	Other nervous disorders
5–9	Pedestrian hit by vehicle	Other nervous disorders
10–14	Pedestrian hit by vehicle	Other nervous disorders
15–19	Motor vehicle accidents	Suicide/undetermined intent by poison
20–24	Motor vehicle accidents	Suicide/undetermined intent by poison
25–29	Suicide/undetermined intent by poison	Motor vehicle accidents
30–34	Breast cancer	Cervical cancer
35–39	Breast cancer	Cervical cancer
40–44	Breast cancer	Cerebrovascular disease
45–49	Breast cancer	Heart attack and chronic heart disease
50–54	Breast cancer	Heart attack and chronic heart disease
55–59	Heart attack and chronic heart disease	Breast cancer
60–64	Heart attack and chronic heart disease	Breast cancer
65–69	Heart attack and chronic heart disease	Cerebrovascular disease
70–74	Heart attack and chronic heart disease	Cerebrovascular disease
75–79	Heart attack and chronic heart disease	Cerebrovascular disease
80–84	Heart attack and chronic heart disease	Cerebrovascular disease
85–89	Heart attack and chronic heart disease	Cerebrovascular disease
90+	Heart attack and chronic heart disease	Pneumonia

Table 5a: Most common and second most common group of death at each age band – males

Males age	Most common group of death	Second most common group of death
0	All respiratory deaths	All deaths due to infections
1–4	All cancer deaths	All respiratory deaths
5–9	All cancer deaths	All transport deaths
10–14	All transport deaths	All cancer deaths
15–19	All transport deaths	All suicide/undetermined deaths
20–24	All transport deaths	All suicide/undetermined deaths
25–29	All suicide/undetermined deaths	All transport deaths
30–34	All suicide/undetermined deaths	All cancer deaths
35–39	All cardiovascular deaths	All cancer deaths
40–44	All cardiovascular deaths	All cancer deaths
45–49	All cardiovascular deaths	All cancer deaths
50–54	All cardiovascular deaths	All cancer deaths
55–59	All cardiovascular deaths	All cancer deaths
60–64	All cardiovascular deaths	All cancer deaths
65–69	All cardiovascular deaths	All cancer deaths
70–74	All cardiovascular deaths	All cancer deaths
75–79	All cardiovascular deaths	All cancer deaths
80–84	All cardiovascular deaths	All cancer deaths
85–89	All cardiovascular deaths	All respiratory deaths
90+	All cardiovascular deaths	All respiratory deaths

Table 5b: Most common and second most common group of death at each age band – females

Females age	Most common group of death	Second most common group of death
0	All respiratory deaths	All deaths due to infections
1–4	All cancer deaths	All respiratory deaths
5–9	All cancer deaths	All transport deaths
10–14	All cancer deaths	All transport deaths
15–19	All transport deaths	All cancer deaths
20–24	All suicide/undetermined deaths	All cancer deaths
25–29	All cancer deaths	All suicide/undetermined deaths
30–34	All cancer deaths	All suicide/undetermined deaths
35–39	All cancer deaths	All cardiovascular deaths
40–44	All cancer deaths	All cardiovascular deaths
45–49	All cancer deaths	All cardiovascular deaths
50–54	All cancer deaths	All cardiovascular deaths
55–59	All cancer deaths	All cardiovascular deaths
60–64	All cancer deaths	All cardiovascular deaths
65–69	All cardiovascular deaths	All cancer deaths
70–74	All cardiovascular deaths	All cancer deaths
75–79	All cardiovascular deaths	All cancer deaths
80–84	All cardiovascular deaths	All cancer deaths
85–89	All cardiovascular deaths	All respiratory deaths
90+	All cardiovascular deaths	All respiratory deaths